C000061204

Other Books By Barbara Trisler

Air Fryer Cookbook For Beginners In 2020

Paleo Diet Cookbook For Diabetics In 2020

<u>Bonus Offer</u>

The kindle edition will be available to you for FREE when you purchase the paperback version

from Amazon.com (The US Store)

Table of Contents

Introduction 7

Chapter 1 8

Insulin And Diabetes 8

The Importance of Insulin 8

How Insulin Controls Your Blood Sugar 9

Chapter 2 11

Type 1 Diabetes 11

What is Type 1 Diabetes? 11

Causes of Type 1 Diabetes Mellitus 11

Symptoms of Type 1 Diabetes 12

When to Visit a Doctor 16

Complications of Type 1 Diabetes 16

Chapter 3 20

Treatment Of Type 1 Diabetes 20

Treatment Method 1 20

Treatment Method 2 22

How to Manage Type 1 Diabetes 22

Things Diabetics Need To Avoided 24

Chapter 4 25

Type 2 Diabetes 25

Type 2 vs. Type 1 Diabetes 25

Causes of Type 2 Diabetes 25

Symptoms of Type 2 Diabetes 26

When to See a Doctor 28

Complications of Type 2 Diabetes 28

Chapter 5 32

Treatment of Type 2 Diabetes 32

Things You Need To Do 34

Things You Need To Avoid 35

Chapter 6 37

Other Types Of Diabetes 37

1. Gestational Diabetes 37

Symptoms of Gestational Diabetes 40

Complications of Gestational Diabetes 40

Some Guidelines for Women with Gestational Diabetes 42

Treatment for Gestational Diabetes 43

Prediabetes 43

Treatment for Prediabetes 44

The Simple Guide

To Diabetes In 2020

A

Helpful Companion To Understanding

Diabetes And its Complications

(Includes Food To Eat & Those To Avoid)

By

Barbara Trisler

www.MillenniumPublishingLimited.com

Copyright ©2020

Disclaimer

This publication is designed to provide competent and reliable information regarding the subject matter covered. However, it is sold with the understanding that the author is not engaged in rendering medical or other professional advice. Laws and practices often vary from state to state and country to country and if medical or other expert assistance is required, the services of a professional should be sought. The author specifically disclaims any liability that is incurred from the use or application of the contents of this book.

Chapter 7 .... **45**

22 Myths About Diabetes **45**

Chapter 8 .... **52**

Prevention & Management Strategy 1 .... **52**

Constant Monitoring 52

How Often Should You Check your Sugar Levels 52

Equipment a Diabetic Should Invest In 53

Chapter 9 .... **56**

Prevention & Management Strategy 2 .... **56**

Attaining and Maintaining A Healthy Weight 56

How to Calculate Your BMI 56

What is the Normal BMI? 57

Weight Loss Guide for Diabetics 57

Ideal Weight Loss Rate for Overweight Diabetics 59

Steps to Correct Weight Loss 60

Maintaining a Healthy Weight 63

Chapter 10 .... **65**

Prevention & Management Strategy 3 .... **65**

Exercise Routines 65

6 Exercise Routines for Diabetics 65

Types Of Exercise To Avoid 66

8 Exercise Safety Measures 67

Chapter 11 .... **70**

Prevention & Management Strategy 4 .... **70**

Diabetic Meal Plans 70

5 Characteristics of a Diabetic Diet 70

How To Calculate Your Daily Carbohydrate, Protein and Fat Requirements (5 Steps) 72

Converting Grams to Calories 73

Getting Macronutrients from the Right Source 74

Types Of Food To Eat & Those To Avoid 75

Distributing your Daily Calorie Needs 78

Recommended schedule of meals 78

Step by Step Guide to Distributing your Calories to Each Meal 79

Chapter 12 .... **84**

Breakfast Recipes For Diabetics **84**

Berry Oatmeal 84

Egg Sandwich 84

Banana Pancakes 85

Apple Quinoa Porridge 86

Vegetable Frittata 87

Lunch and Dinner Recipes **89**

Pan-Fried Tuna with Pineapple Salsa 89

Broiled Salmon with Brown Rice..90

Beef and Vegetable Stir Fry 90

Chicken Whole-Wheat Pasta 91

Low-Fat Chicken Tenders...92

Macronutrient Conversion Table **94**

Conclusion.. **97**

The End **98**

Introduction

In November 2016, the World Health Organization (WHO) published new statistics regarding diabetes. The number of people diagnosed with the condition has increased from the 108 million reported in 1980, to more than 400 million in 2014. In 2012 alone, around 1.5 million deaths were directly attributed to diabetes. WHO projects that by 2030, diabetes will be the seventh leading cause of death.

The statistics may warrant calling diabetes a global epidemic. Worse, many people are still unaware of what diabetes is.

Many patients diagnosed with diabetes only start to look up information, regarding diabetes, after they are diagnosed. Also, studies show that by the time a patient is diagnosed with diabetes, it is likely the disease has already caused secondary conditions, such as kidney disease or eye damage. Prescribed treatments, to reverse or control diabetes, can also cause other organs to be affected and new conditions to arise.

This guide is designed to educate the average reader, with regards to diabetes. If they have already been diagnosed; they can learn to manage the condition. It can even help you try and prevent diabetes occurring in the first place.

The book is divided into two parts. The first part discusses the types of diabetes, their symptoms, complications and differences. A chapter is also dedicated to exposing the myths regarding diabetes.

The second part discusses how to prevent and manage diabetes. It outlines the steps you should take to lose weight; and other things that can help to avoid, prevent, or manage various types of diabetes. There are also recipes for diabetics and a handy table to help you keep track of your calorie intake.

I hope this book, will help guide you to deal with diabetes and how to protect yourself from the condition.

Chapter 1

Insulin And Diabetes

It is difficult to give a precise definition of the word "diabetes," because there is more than one type. For example, there is Diabetes Insipidus, a condition characterized by heightened thirst and dilute urine. Pre-diabetes is a condition where your sugar level tends to be higher than normal after fasting—The medical term is impaired fasting glucose. The sugar level can also be higher after eating—The medical term for this, is impaired glucose tolerance. Gestational Diabetes refers to the type that can occur during pregnancy.

However, when most people say "diabetes", they are likely to be referring to Diabetes Mellitus, which is the condition typified by a high blood sugar level. This is a metabolic condition, where the body does not produce the correct level of insulin, or does not respond to the insulin produced, and causes the level of glucose in the blood to increase.

Thus, for this guide, we will use the term "diabetes" to refer to diabetes mellitus, unless specified otherwise.

The Importance of Insulin

The one common factor, in every type of diabetes, is the function of the hormone, insulin. It is responsible for how your body stores and uses the glucose obtained from the carbohydrates you eat.

Insulin is produced in the pancreas, in what are called beta cells. These cells primary function is to store and release insulin into the bloodstream. The beta cells respond to an increase in the amount of glucose in the blood stream, by secreting insulin.

Glucose is needed by the body, as it is can easily break it down for energy use. A person with low levels of glucose in their bloodstream may feel lethargic, dizzy, and their muscles may shake. However, a person with high amounts of glucose in their bloodstream may experience: blurred vision, a frequent urge to urinate, severe thirst, anxiety, muscle tingling, and fatigue.

Having an abnormally low or high level of glucose in your bloodstream is dangerous. Having a low amount of glucose may cause your body and brain to shut down; while too much glucose may be toxic.

A healthy body produces insulin, to ensure there is just enough glucose in the bloodstream for it to function on any given day. The amount a person requires, varies according to their daily physical activity. An athlete or a person that exercises regularly may need more glucose. A person who is not as active will need less glucose.

How Insulin Controls Your Blood Sugar

Understanding how insulin affects your blood sugar level, will enable you to understand the different types of diabetes mellitus. Insulin works to control the glucose in the body in the following way:

1. When a person eats something, it is digested by their stomach and subsequently passes through the small intestine. Here, it is broken down by enzymes into small sugar units, one of which is glucose.

2. The glucose is absorbed by the blood vessels in the small intestine. It is then transported to the cells, or parts of the body that need it, such as the brain or muscle tissue. However, the body does not use all the glucose obtained from food. It also stores some of the glucose in various parts of the body i.e. the liver, fat and muscle cells. This is especially the case if a person is not physically active, or their activity is restricted in some way e.g. illness.

3. The body releases insulin, to control the amount of glucose stored in these cells. This process happens, when blood passes through the pancreas. The pancreas releases the beta cells; and if the cells realize there is too much glucose circulating in the body, it will release a proportionate amount of insulin to convert the glucose into a form that can be stored. It will not release insulin, if the amount of glucose is low.

Without insulin, the human body cannot use glucose or store it for energy. As a result, the glucose stays in the bloodstream, causing harmful side effects.

There are two types of Diabetes. We will go into greater detail, regarding Type 1 and Type 2 diabetes, in the following chapters.

Chapter 2

Type 1 Diabetes

Type 1 Diabetes used to be called "Juvenile Diabetes," because the symptoms usually manifest during adolescence. However, if you look at recent statistics, you will notice even adults develop type 1 diabetes. With this condition, the patient usually requires insulin injections to regulate the level of glucose in their body.

What is Type 1 Diabetes?

Type 1 diabetes is a chronic condition, where the pancreas does not produce enough insulin for the body's needs.

Remember, in the body of a healthy person, the pancreas contains beta cells that recognize when adequate glucose has been released into specific cells and trigger the action of insulin.

A person with type 1 diabetes has a pancreas with no functioning beta cells. When they consume something with a high sugar or carbohydrate content, the food is broken down into glucose, but when the glucose passes through the pancreas, there are no beta cells to trigger the production of insulin. This means no insulin "guides" the glucose to enter cells to help them function; or for storage. The excess glucose is not stored in the fat and muscle cells, or liver – it will instead remain in the bloodstream.

Causes of Type 1 Diabetes Mellitus

There are two possible causes of type 1 diabetes. The most common is an autoimmune disease, that prevents the cells from producing insulin. The second, is an acquired disease that causes the pancreas to malfunction.

Type 1 Diabetes Mellitus, as an Autoimmune Disease

An autoimmune disease is a disorder that causes your immune system to malfunction. It is unable to recognize healthy cells, and mistakenly identifies them as foreign invaders. The body then proceeds to destroy them, which can cause great harm to various tissue, structures and organs.

Type 1 diabetes may be caused by an autoimmune disorder, where your body refuses to recognize the beta cells as "good cells." Your immune system attacks them, and renders them incapable of producing insulin. Without the insulin, the levels of glucose in the bloodstream continues to rise and eventually becomes toxic.

Type 1 Diabetes Mellitus, as an Acquired Disease

This second type of diabetes is rare. Type 1 diabetes is rarely acquired, but when it is, it is usually due to a physical event that affects the pancreas, such as pancreatic cancer or an accident that causes injury to the pancreas.

The pancreas fails to create enough beta cells required to produce a sufficient amount of insulin for the body's requirements.

Symptoms of Type 1 Diabetes

The symptoms of type 1 diabetes and type 2 diabetes are similar. The difference is, that symptoms of type 1 diabetes usually manifest at an earlier age.

1. Frequent urination

2. Excessive thirst

3. Bedwetting

4. Easily tired or exhausted

5. Sleepy

6. Extreme hunger

7. Blurred vision

8. Vaginal yeast infection (Thrush)

9. Weight loss or difficulty gaining weight

However, these symptoms may not always be due to Type 1 diabetes. They may be caused by another disease or condition. Hence, for the symptoms to be indicative of diabetes, the following conditions must be met:

- Sudden onset—The person has not experienced the symptoms before. They did not do, or experience any physical activity that may have caused it.

- After the first appearance of a symptom, it persists.

- Two or more symptoms on the list are present.

1. Frequent Urination

To illustrate:

> Your child wets the bed for the first time, and they did not take any diuretic medication that could have caused it. You note that it has occurred multiple times in a week. He is also sleepy a lot of the time.
>
> In the above example, the child's bedwetting *may* be a symptom of Type 1 diabetes.
>
> If, however, your child is given a diuretic every day, for 7 days and they wet the bed during those 7 nights. However, when they stop taking the medication, the bedwetting stops. This is not likely to be caused by Type 1 diabetes, even if they tend to be sleepy most of the time.

- The symptoms had manifested before the patient reached the age of 20.

2. Excessive Thirst

On average, an adult may urinate up to 8 to 10 times a day, while a child may urinate 10 to 14 times a day. If the number of times you urinate exceeds the average by 20%, then it may be considered frequent. Therefore, if an adult urinates upwards of 12 times a day and the child urinates 16 to 18 times a day, this would be considered frequency.

Other evidence is of frequency is when a person wakes during the night, just to urinate. According to studies, when we sleep, the body regulates our system. If we wake to urinate then there may be something wrong.

How to tell if thirst is excessive

Normally, a child will only drink one glass of water whenever they are thirsty and an adult may drink one to two glasses of water. This amount is enough to quench normal thirst. However, if the child or adult frequently drink more than this, without any obvious reason (e.g. running around or working out,) they may be suffering from excessive thirst, due to diabetes mellitus.

N.B: There are many reasons a person may become excessively thirsty. They may be suffering from dehydration due to the summer heat or because of physical activity. In the absence of any obvious reasons, excessive thirst may be a symptom of a medical condition such as diabetes.

3. Blurred Vision

For blurred vision to become a symptom of diabetes, it must be frequent and not continuous. If the blurred vision is continuous, it may be a symptom of eye disorder or disease. If you frequently experience blurred vision, which comes and goes, it may be a sign of degeneration, which can be a complication of diabetes.

4. Exhaustion, Fatigue and Sleepiness

Exhaustion, fatigue and sleepiness are common for any person who experiences strenuous physical activity. However, if the person gets adequate sleep and rest, but is still tired and sleepy, it may be a symptom of diabetes.

5. Extreme Hunger

Hunger is considered extreme when a person eats a *full meal, every two hours;* and this hunger occurs for several days. If they eat more than usual just for a day, it would not be considered extreme hunger.

Extreme and unusual hunger, as a symptom of diabetes, occurs because your body cells do not receive glucose, therefore *no signal is sent to your brain to tell you you're full*. Your brain still thinks you are depriving yourself of food.

6. Sudden Weight Loss or Difficulty Gaining Weight

Weight loss can be considered sudden, if the person loses more than ten percent of their weight in a month. This is without being on a weight loss diet, or engaging in any weight loss activity.

A person is defined as having difficulty gaining weight, if they cannot reach their ideal weight, despite eating food that has a high-fat content or observing a weight-gain diet.

This is again attributed to the failure of the cells to send signals to certain organs, due to a lack of glucose. Your body does not give the signal to your liver, to release fat cells that help you gain or lose weight. In addition, it doesn't tell your body to develop more muscles cells to tone your body.

When to Visit a Doctor

You need to visit your doctor or specialist, if at least two of the symptoms described are present. Tests should be considered, particularly a urinalysis and a fasting blood sugar (FBS) test.

If the results of the tests are abnormal, you will need to make another appointment to see the doctor for interpretation, professional diagnoses and additional testing.

As a parent, if you notice sudden weight loss, extreme tiredness or weakness in your child, make sure to visit your pediatrician immediately. The doctor may order a fasting blood sugar on your child, further tests and examinations.

Complications of Type 1 Diabetes

With type 1 diabetes, the body is almost completely unable to produce insulin, whereas in type 2 diabetes, the body is merely experiencing insulin resistance. With insulin resistance, the body can still produce insulin, but the body cannot utilize it efficiently.

During the early part of the twentieth century, if a person was diagnosed with type 1 diabetes, they were only given a life expectancy of one year. The disease itself, was not necessarily what shortened their lifespan. However, the complications that arose from the diabetes were.

Below are some complications of Type 1 diabetes. A few also occur in Type 2 Diabetes:

Ketoacidosis

Due to a lack of insulin, the cells do not receive enough glucose to fuel the body. The body then must convert stored fat into energy, to compensate for the lack of glucose. However, this causes the liver to release ketones.

High levels of ketones in the body can cause complications, ranging from minor to severe. In fact, most symptoms of diabetes are due to ketoacidosis.

The effects of ketoacidosis:

1. Frequent urination

2. Extreme thirst

3. Cold skin

4. Confusion

5. Abdominal pain

6. Fruity breath

Ketoacidosis is a serious symptom, and needs prompt emergency treatment, if a person is vomiting; can't tolerate food or liquid, and has a blood sugar level of more than 300mg/dl or 16.7 mmol/L.

According to statistics, ketoacidosis occurs more frequently in people with type 1 diabetes, than those with type II diabetes.

Neuropathy

This is more commonly known as nerve damage. High amounts of glucose in the blood may damage the nerves in the body's system. Nerves send signals to organs in the body, triggering them to react. If they are damaged, then these signals can be broken or disrupted. This may result in numbness, or loss of sensation, then pain and weakness may follow.

Neuropathy usually starts with the nerves in the feet. The person may experience tingling and could lose sensation. They may not be able to feel when their feet are injured or irritated, thus making them more prone to infection.

This complication may also target other parts of the body, such as the wrists or ankles, can limit the use of the affected part, and in extreme cases cause paralysis.

It can also target the inner organs of the body, which make it hard for them to control their automatic reactions. An example of this is bedwetting, where the person's bladder does not receive the signal, to prevent them urinating whilst asleep.

Retinopathy

This is a microvascular complication of diabetes. The retinas are the part of our eyes that traps light, enabling us to see things around us. The light signals our optic nerve, so the latter can interpret what we are seeing.

Blood travels to the retinas in the eyes; but if there is a high amount of glucose present in the blood, the retinas may be damaged. When the retina is damaged, loss of vision may occur.

Nephropathy

Other organs that may be damaged, due to a high level of glucose, are the kidneys. The kidneys act as a filter, separating toxins from the bloodstream. They produce liters of water, in the form of urine, to flush out these toxins. However, they are also responsible for distributing calcium and protein to other organs and producing hemoglobin for red blood cells.

The kidneys recognize the excess glucose in the bloodstream as a toxin, and therefore push the glucose out. If the level of glucose in the blood is constantly high, the kidneys must work harder and longer to flush the glucose out. This causes an affected person to urinate more frequently.

If the glucose level continues to rise, our kidneys will only focus on filtering it out of the blood, and "forget" about their other functions. The kidneys may become overworked, which may lead to nephropathy.

Heart Disease

High glucose levels in the blood can also result in heart disease. The excess glucose causes plaque to build up in the walls of the arteries and veins of the heart. The veins become clogged and the heart must work harder, to pump blood around the body's system.

The heart will begin to weaken; and as it weakens, the person may suffer complications, such as hypertension (high blood pressure) or a cerebral vascular accident (stroke.)

Books By Barbara Trisler	
Book #	**Book Title**
1	Air Fryer Cookbook For Beginners
2	Air Fryer Cookbook For Beginners With Colour Pictures
3	Paleo Diet Cookbook For Diabetics
4	Paleo Diet Cookbook For Diabetics With Colour Pictures
5	Air Fryer Cookbook For Beginners (2nd Edition)
The kindle edition will be available to you for FREE when you purchase the paperback version from Amazon.com (The US Store)	

Chapter 3

Treatment Of Type 1 Diabetes

Thankfully, the life expectancy of those with type 1 diabetes has now been extended. However, it is still on average, eleven years less than a non-diabetic person. The extension in life expectancy, is attributed to pharmaceutical and medical breakthroughs, that have led to the discovery of more effective treatments for type 1 diabetes.

Today, there are two recognized treatments for type 1 diabetes:

Treatment Method 1

Insulin injections

This is the most common treatment for type 1 diabetes. Insulin is injected by the person, to help regulate their blood sugar levels. However, the effect of insulin is short-term, and as the disease progresses, they may require higher dosages of insulin to control their blood sugar.

Insulin injections are also not always successful in preventing the complications of diabetes.

Possible side effects of Insulin Injections

Hypoglycemia

Insulin injections can pose dangerous side-effects, if they are not administered and monitored correctly. An overdose of insulin may result in hypoglycemia, where the person's blood glucose drops too low.

It is easy to recover from the effects of hypoglycemia. The patient needs to consume food or drink that contains a high level of sugar e.g. candies, soda etc. However, if hypoglycemia is not treated immediately, it may lead to severe and life-threatening complications.

Below are the signs and symptoms that may suggest a person is suffering from hypoglycemia:

- Excessive sweating

- Arrhythmia or rapid heartbeat

- Paleness

- Slurred speech

- Anxiety

- Poor cognition skills

- Sleepiness

Another danger with insulin is ketoacidosis. The sudden introduction of insulin into the body, during ketoacidosis, may cause the blood sugar to plummet, which may result in hypoglycaemia. The sudden drop in sugar level may cause cerebral edema, which could cause the person to lose consciousness. It can even lead to coma or in the most severe cases, death.

Hyperglycemia

This is caused when too much glucose is present in the blood stream. Temporary hyperglycemia is not an issue. However, if the condition becomes chronic, it can lead to other complications e.g. kidney, heart or retinal damage. Neuropathy may even occur. Treatment aims to keep blood sugar levels as close to normal, to avoid long term complications. This involves diet, exercise and medication.

Acute hyperglycemia, involving extremely high sugar levels, is a medical emergency. It may rapidly cause severe complications, for example fluid loss. It is more common in insulin dependent diabetics, that are uncontrolled.

Hyperglycemia can be a serious problem, if not treated in time. In untreated hyperglycemia, ketoacidosis can occur. Ketoacidosis develops when the body does not have enough insulin. Without insulin, the body can't utilize the glucose for fuel, so the body starts to break down fats for energy.

Ketoacidosis is a life-threatening condition that needs immediate treatment. Symptoms include: shortness of breath, breath that smells fruity, nausea and vomiting, and very dry mouth. Chronic hyperglycemia injures the heart of patients and is also associated with heart attacks and death in people that have no previous history of heart disease or heart failure.

Treatment Method 2

Pancreas Transplant

Type 1 diabetes is due to a defective pancreas. If a healthier pancreas is transplanted into the body, it may be able to produce the insulin required and the person would no longer need insulin injections.

Many people hope a transplant will be *the* cure. However, this option is usually only recommended by doctors and experts, if insulin injections do not successfully control blood glucose levels. A pancreas transplant may cure type 1 diabetes permanently, but it can come with its own risks and complications.

According to studies, the body naturally prefers its native pancreas. If it is substituted with a new one, the risk of rejection is high. The patient's life may be in danger, if this occurs.

How to Manage Type 1 Diabetes

Aside from insulin injections, there are certain things a type 1 diabetic needs to amend in their lifestyle, to avoid complications. Here are a few dos and don'ts.

- ***Get the right amount of sleep***

  The correct amount of sleep is important for everyone. However, if a Type 1 diabetic does not get the correct amount of sleep, complications can arise.

  N.B: It needs to be "the correct amount of sleep." A diabetic person should not sleep for too long a period, as it increases the risk of hypoglycemia. Blood sugar levels tend to drop, when the body is at rest.

It is dangerous if a person's blood sugar level becomes critically low, while they are asleep. The body may not send signals to the patient's brain to wake up. This may lead to life-threatening situations, like a coma.

If a person does not get enough sleep, they may suffer from hyperglycemia (high blood sugar), as the blood circulates faster when a person is awake. Though not as dangerous as hypoglycemia, it may still be life threatening.

Experts suggest that a type 1 diabetic should not exceed 7 hours of sleep, but not less than 5 hours. They may take some short duration naps during the day, but they should not exceed an hour, or the diabetic may be left feeling more tired.

- **_Exercise_**

    This may be a difficult task for a type I diabetic as they can easily tire, but it is necessary. Type 1 diabetics should exercise more, if they want to lower the amount of insulin they require. Physical activity helps to process carbohydrates or glucose, so the more a person exercises, the less insulin they will require. Exercise also helps improve your body's sensitivity to insulin, as a person burns calories doing physical activity,

- **_Observe a balanced diet_**

    Since a type 1 diabetic cannot process glucose effectively, it is only logical that they should lower their sugar intake. Experts agree, that regardless of the nature of the person's diet, they should be mindful of their carbohydrates and sugar intake.

    It is recommended that diabetics eat small meals, every 2 to 3 hours, instead of eating large meals every 4 to 6 hours. This way, the glucose consumed is at a constant level. This limits the chance of experiencing hypoglycemic or hyperglycemic attacks.

    Veganism and vegetarianism, may not be an appropriate diet for a type 1 diabetic, as they may require more nutritional value than can be found in veganism and vegetarianism. Regardless, it is recommended that all diabetics visit a nutritionist to help them tailor a suitable diet plan. Unlike Type 2 diabetics, type 1 diabetics have more difficulty gaining weight than losing it.

Things Diabetics Need To Avoided

- ***Skipping meals and eating large meals***

  Skipping meals is dangerous for a type 1 diabetic. Their body does not have the required glucose reserves. If they skip meals, they can deprive themselves of the glucose needed to remain healthy, and it could result in hypoglycemia.

  Experts suggest that all diabetics, regardless of type, eat within an hour of waking.

  Eating large meals should also be avoided, as it can cause a type 1 diabetic to have a spike in their glucose levels, which may result in hyperglycemia.

- ***Eating high sugar and refined foods***

  A type 1 diabetic cannot convert sugar into energy. Eating high-sugar foods will increase their blood sugar levels, and without counteracting this with insulin, it may become dangerous.

  In addition, if their blood sugar level drops suddenly, after consuming high sugar foods, damage may occur in the veins and can even cause cerebral edema.

- ***Not monitoring the blood sugar regularly***

  For a type 1 diabetic, testing their blood glucose level should be done at least six times a day. It is usually tested after waking in the morning, before meals and before you sleep at night.

  Blood glucose monitoring is more important for type 1 diabetics, than type 2 diabetics. This is due to the complications that a sudden change in blood glucose level might cause.

Chapter 4

Type 2 Diabetes

Type 2 diabetes is a chronic metabolic disorder, caused by resistance in the cells to the insulin produced by the body. This causes glucose to remain in the bloodstream.

A person who has a fasting blood sugar level of more than 6.4mmol/L or a routine blood sugar level of 11mmol/L is considered to have type 2 diabetes, especially if it is accompanied by symptoms of this type.

Type 2 vs. Type 1 Diabetes

Remember how insulin helps break down glucose into energy, i.e. that is what occurs in non-diabetics. In Type 1 diabetes, the body does not produce insulin or produces significantly less insulin that is needed by the body. However, in type 2 diabetes, this is what happens:

1. Glucose passes through the pancreas and triggers the beta cells to produce insulin.
2. The body does not have a problem producing insulin. The insulin carries out its role and directs glucose to the cells, including fat and muscle cells.
3. However, in type 2 diabetes, the cells resist the insulin and refuse to accept the glucose. Alternatively, there is an agent present in the cell, which refuses to recognize the insulin, keeping it and the glucose out of the cell. The glucose does not go directly to the cells.
4. Glucose is pushed back into the bloodstream and remains there, until external intervention e.g. medication.

In type 1 diabetes, the cell does not absorb the glucose; therefore the organs are unable to function due to a lack of fuel. In type 2 diabetes, some glucose may still make it inside the cells, although the energy acquired may not be enough to make the organ function correctly.

Causes of Type 2 Diabetes

The cause of type 2 diabetes is lifestyle and genetics. The following may increase a person's risk of acquiring type 2 diabetes:

a.   Consuming a lot of carbohydrates and simple sugars

b.   Low physical activity, or a sedentary lifestyle

c.   Being overweight or obese

d.   Hormonal imbalance, that results in an abnormal increase in appetite

e.   Having direct relatives with a history of diabetes e.g. Mother or Father

Why do these factors lead to Type 2 Diabetes?

These factors, except for genetics, can cause cells to be required to process too much glucose.

Imagine a pizza delivery guy, who delivers pizza for free. Every minute, he delivers a pizza to your house. Perhaps, for the first dozen boxes, you still get excited, because pizza is great. However, after a few dozen more, you would tell the pizza guy to stop delivering.

If he continues to deliver, you will stop opening the door to him, so he would send the pizza to your neighbors. But, your neighbor has been receiving the same amount of pizza and refused to accept it. The pizza guy would have no choice but to find a place to deliver the pizza. The pizza may become rotten and toxic, before he can find a new recipient, and when they eventually receive it, it causes them harm.

This is the exact relationship between your cells and glucose. Your cells receive too much glucose because of a high sugar intake. Therefore, it closes its doors and forces your body to find a new place for the glucose. This high level of glucose remains in your bloodstream, and it becomes toxic. When it travels to other organs, like your liver and kidneys, it harms them. This is when complications start to arise.

Symptoms of Type 2 Diabetes

The symptoms of type 2 diabetes are almost the same as Type 1 diabetes. However, how the symptoms develop and progress differ:

1. In type 2 diabetes, the symptoms usually start to manifest upwards of the age of thirty. Whereas, in type 1 diabetes, the symptoms start as early as at 7 years old.

2. The symptoms of type 2 diabetes occur gradually. While on the other hand, the symptoms of type 1 diabetes, as mentioned before, are sudden and are easier to identify. This is the reason a type 2 diabetic discovers the disease later in life. Statistics show, that type 2 diabetics are routinely diagnosed five to ten years after the initial symptoms have occurred.

Symptoms of Type 2 Diabetes, that are Rarely Present in Type 1 Diabetes

Due to the delayed onset of type 2 diabetes, symptoms may be present that are rarely seen in type 1 diabetes.

a. **Acanthosis Nigricans (dark patches)**

Dark patches can be present around the neck, the underarms, and other parts of the body. This is due to insulin resistance and the skin's inability to control the production of melanin.

However, many experts suggest acanthosis nigricans may be a coincidental symptom, as many type 2 diabetics are obese. Obesity often causes the folds in the skin to become darker.

b. **Hair Loss or Thinning**

New studies show that hair loss, or thinning, may be an indication of type 2 diabetes. The hair follicles weaken and new ones develop slower, due to a lack of fuel in the cells. This symptom is more visible in females than males.

When to See a Doctor

As with type 1 diabetes, having two or more of the symptoms should be evidence enough for your doctor to arrange a blood glucose test. However, anyone over the age of thirty is advised to have a *regular urine test* for sugar, even if there are no symptoms of diabetes.

Abnormal values in sugar level, both in the fasting blood sugar test and a urine test should be followed up by further tests.

Complications of Type 2 Diabetes

It is somewhat true that, when it comes to complications, all types of diabetes are the same. The complications, that result from type 2 diabetes, are the same as for type 1 diabetes. However, their development is slower.

In fact, in early twentieth century, diagnosis of type 2 diabetes was not common. Patients were not diagnosed with diabetes, as the symptoms were diagnosed differently - as many were unassociated with diabetes.

According to experts, the complications of type 2 diabetes are preventable and reversible. The progress of these complications is gradual; and doctors often treat them, before they become worse.

Below are complications of Type 2 diabetes and how their progress differs from Type 1.

1. **Ketoacidosis**

   Type 2 diabetics may experience mild ketoacidosis, and unlike type 1 diabetes, ketoacidosis does not develop within twenty-four hours. Type 2 diabetics may only experience minor symptoms of ketoacidosis, when their blood sugar level is significantly higher than 17mmol/L.

2. **Microvascular eye disease**

Retinopathy is not common for type 2 diabetics. However, they are still prone to eye damages and disease, such as blurred vision and cataracts. If the patient has a history of glaucoma, their risk is doubled if they are diagnosed with type 2 diabetes.

3. Hearing Impairment

Diabetic patients may suffer from ear damage, if they do not control their blood sugar levels. However, the risk of hearing impairment with type 2 diabetes is higher. The reason, according to some experts, is that patients with type 2 diabetes acquire the disease at an older age. Their nerves are weaker and are more easily damaged by sudden fluctuations in blood sugar levels.

4. Neuropathy

The nerve damage, caused by type 2 diabetes, is gradual. They rarely develop more serious neuropathy like mononeuropathy and automatic neuropathy. Most type 2 diabetics only suffer peripheral neuropathy, which is usually the loss of sensation in their feet and legs.

5. Nephropathy

Type 2 diabetics may suffer from nephropathy, but it is not as uncontrollable as for type 1 diabetics.

In type 2 diabetes, the level of glucose in the blood fluctuates but rarely exceeds 17mmol/l, which is considered a dangerous level. The negative effect of glucose, on the kidneys, is milder so, it takes longer for them to fail. Also, the level of glucose is lower, the kidneys can continue to carry out their other functions.

6. Heart Disease

Some experts do not believe that type 2 diabetes causes heart disease. They maintain that the heart disease develops alongside diabetes.

Type 2 diabetes can be triggered by passive lifestyle. The person may develop it because they are obese, physically inactive and eating high levels of carbohydrate. This lifestyle can also trigger heart disease.

However, research shows type 2 diabetes causes deterioration of the heart muscle, as it will increase the amount of plaque in the artery. This means the heart muscles will need to generate more pressure in order to move blood through those clogged up arteries. Also, it makes it difficult for the body to reduce excess cholesterol, which increases the risk of heart disease.

7. Slow Healing of wounds

Wound infection can be a far more serious complication in type 2 diabetes. *Type 2 diabetic patients have slower healing than type 1 diabetic patients.* In type 2 diabetes, the cells refuse to accept glucose, which is the source of energy required, to multiply and repair tissue. Therefore, patients' wounds heal more slowly and become at risk of infection. In type 1 diabetes, the cells may receive the correct dose of glucose, when the patient has a sufficient insulin supply.

8. Skin pigmentation and irritation

Studies show that hyperglycemia may cause skin complications. However, because the cells of type 2 diabetics refuse to accept glucose, the skin doesn't produce enough keratin. Their skin is usually rough, dull, dry and at risk of skin pigmentation and irritation.

9. Dental Decay and Gum Disease

Diabetics are more prone to dental decay and gum disease. However, type 2 diabetics are at a higher risk, because the gum muscles weaken due to insulin resistance. It also makes the mouth more prone to infections.

Also, if the person suffers from ketoacidosis, his/her teeth will weaken due to the acidity in the mouth.

10. **Hyperglycemic Hyperosmolar Nonketotic Syndrome (HHNS)**

Patients with either type of diabetes may experience this condition. It is life threatening and may prove fatal if not treated within a few hours.

It occurs when the level of sugar in the blood reaches upwards of 33mmol/L. Severe ketoacidosis and neuropathy may occur and cause: Weakness, fever - above 101^0F, extreme thirst, hallucination, dark or murky urine, and drowsiness.

If you suspect you, or someone else, has this condition, go to the emergency room immediately, as treatment is critical.

N.B. Forcing the sudden drop of the person's glucose level, may result in other life-threatening conditions.

11. **Erectile dysfunction**

This is where a man either cannot have an erection, or cannot maintain an erection for sufficient time, to have sexual intercourse. Uncontrolled blood sugar, whether for type 1 or type 2 diabetes, may result in erectile dysfunction. This is due to the small blood vessels easily rupturing following an erection. Also, the nerves surrounding the penis can be affected.

12. **Vaginal itching**

Women with type 2 diabetes may suffer from vaginal dryness, which can result in vaginal itching. The itching occurs on the labia and even on their thighs. It is caused by the presence of sugar in the urine. If the woman does not maintain a sufficient level of hygiene, she may develop vaginitis or a yeast infection (thrush.)

Chapter 5

Treatment of Type 2 Diabetes

There is no available cure for Type 2 diabetes. However, it can be managed, by medication and a change in lifestyle.

Medication

Doctors often prescribe two types of medication for type 2 diabetes. There are medications that increase the sensitivity of your body's cells to insulin and medications that lower the blood glucose level. The following is a list of the most commonly prescribed medication.

1. Metformin

This is the first and primary medication to be prescribed to a pre diabetic or a type 2 diabetic. This drug aims to increase the sensitivity of the body to insulin - it engages the cells and encourages them to accept glucose.

There are certain side effects of metformin. Pharmaceutical companies claim nausea and diarrhea are possible side effects of metformin. Some patients also claim loss of appetite, but experts relate this to nausea and diarrhea. The body needs time to adjust to the effects of metformin, and the side effects may eventually disappear.

Some studies claim that metformin plays a significant role in increasing the risk of kidney disease, among patients.

2. Thiazolidinedione

This drug works in a similar way to metformin, but has a faster and stronger effect. It also has more serious side effects than metformin.

Thiazolidinedione promotes weight gain. It may also trigger an increase in fat storage, in the body, which could lead to heart failure and other associated disease. It has also been claimed, that it lowers calcium levels in the body, which increases the risk of osteoporosis and bone fracture.

This drug is only prescribed to type 2 diabetics, with blood sugar levels that exceed 20mmol/L.

3. Sulfonylureas.

Sulfonylureas aim to control blood sugar levels, by triggering the pancreas to produce more insulin. The body requires insulin to counteract the glucose in the blood. A high amount of insulin can force the cells to recognize it and accept the glucose.

The side effects of sulfonylureas include: weight gain, an increase in appetite and sudden hypoglycemia. It is recommended they be taken fifteen to thirty minutes before meals, to lessen the side effects.

4. Meglitinides

These drugs are like sulfonylureas, but cause blood sugar levels to drop faster. Unlike sulfonylureas, the effect of meglitinides is temporary. A patient would take this if their blood sugar level suddenly rose above 20mmol/L.

Taking meglitinides, with a blood sugar level lower than 16mmol/L, may result in hypoglycemia.

Like sulfonylureas, meglitinides also increases appetite, which may lead to weight gain. However, doctors would normally prescribe meglitinides for short periods.

Other Methods of Managing Type 2 Diabetes

In addition to the drugs mentioned, there have been recent medical breakthroughs that can help control type 2 diabetes:

Inhibitors

This medication lowers the blood sugar level by decreasing the absorption of glucose. Some inhibitors coat the digestive system, with a substance that blocks sugar or carbohydrates, and force them out as urine. Others trigger the kidneys to expel glucose, as they filter it.

Inhibitors are not good at lowering blood sugar levels, but are good at controlling the fluctuation of the levels. However, because they flush out sugar in the urine, the patient may become prone to urinary tract infections and yeast infections. Some women may suffer stickiness in their vaginal area.

Insulin therapy

A few decades ago, doctors refused to give insulin injections to type 2 diabetics, as they did not believe they would have an effect. However, it has been discovered that during the early stage of the disease, taking insulin injections can slow the progression and boost the sensitivity of the cells to insulin.

Things You Need To Do

Managing Type 2 diabetes is the same as Type 1 diabetes.

Type 2 diabetic patients need to:

- Get sufficient sleep

- Exercise

- Eating a balanced diet

Things You Need To Avoid

1. **Eating too high a carbohydrate and fat diet, in relation to your physical activity**

   People with type 1 diabetes should not eat foods that have high carbohydrates, but they may eat more fat. Their bodies do not produce insulin and can't convert sugar into energy. Their body converts fats into energy instead. Whereas, type 2 diabetics, should eat a diet with a balanced carbohydrate to fat ratio.

   One cause of type 2 diabetes is obesity. The patient should lower their body fat index, to make their cells more sensitive to insulin.

   Their diet should be in proportion to the amount of physical activity they do. If the patient is active, then they can eat more carbohydrate and healthy fats. If they are passive, then they should eat less.

2. **Eating or drinking food in large quantities**

   Type 2 diabetics usually have an increased appetite, during meal times. The sudden influx of sugar during meal times, can rapidly increase the blood sugar level. This may trigger hyperglycemia, which increases the risk of complications in other organs of the body.

   Eating five times a day, in small portions, is preferable to eating three times a day, in large portions.

3. **Taking comfort in eating sweet foods**

   Sweets and chocolate help us release happy hormones. However, people with type 2 diabetes, or those previously diagnosed with gestational diabetes, should avoid eating too many sweets and chocolate. There are better ways to release happy hormones, than eating sugar. For example, they could try working out a bit.

4. Becoming stressed

Stress is proven to increase the resistance of insulin in type 2 diabetes. It also encourages people to eat sweet foods. People with increased levels of stress, often forget to eat on time or ignore the complications of diabetes. This can lead to more serious complications. Doctors suggest diabetics get sufficient rest and activity to help them unwind.

Chapter 6

Other Types Of Diabetes

These types of diabetes are temporary and reversible. However, failure to control them can lead to complications. They may even develop into more serious condition most likely, type 2 diabetes.

1. Gestational Diabetes

Gestational diabetes affects pregnant women. According to recent surveys, eleven per cent of pregnant women, around the world, suffer from gestational diabetes; and this is more prevalent in women of Asian descent.

Cause of Gestational Diabetes and Who Are at Risk

When a woman is pregnant, she needs a higher dose of insulin because she must provide glucose to the unborn baby. Her own body may become insulin resistant due to hormonal imbalance during pregnancy.

In normal situations, the baby resolves this as it receives the excess glucose. However, if the baby is also insulin resistant, it will not receive enough glucose for it's needs. The excess glucose the baby cannot absorb returns to the mother, causing her blood glucose levels to rise.

Women with the following characteristics have a higher risk of developing gestational diabetes:

a. Between the age of twenty-five and forty-five years old

b. A normal weight before pregnancy

c. Parents that have a history of diabetes

d. Did not eat an excess of sugary food, prior to pregnancy

e. Previously gave birth to a baby weighing more than eight pounds

f. If they were born with the disorder, macrosomia.

Those who are between twenty-five to forty-five years old

A woman *under thirty years* of age, but *over twenty-five*, has a higher chance of her diabetes being gestational diabetes, unless a problem with her pancreas is discovered.

Type 1 diabetic patients are normally diagnosed before the age of twenty. So, unless the pregnant woman has developed a disease in her pancreas, there is no reason she would produce less or no amount of insulin.

Type 2 diabetic patients experience symptoms at age thirty and over. So, if the pregnant woman is below that age, her diabetes may only be gestational diabetes.

However, if a pregnant woman develops high blood sugar, when she was over thirty years, her diabetes will not be declared gestational, unless it is properly investigated.

A normal weight before pregnancy

Pregnancy can cause sudden hormonal imbalances in women. The hormones may trigger an increase in appetite and weight gain, which could even be borderline obesity. The body automatically defends itself from this sudden imbalance, by making the cells resistant to insulin.

Parents that have a history of diabetes

Diabetes is hereditary. A person who has at least one diabetic parent has a higher risk of acquiring the disease. If the pregnant woman is over thirty years old and her parent or parents have diabetes, she should be investigated thoroughly, before ruling out chronic diabetes.

If she is below thirty and one or both of her parents have a history of diabetes, there is a higher chance the diabetes is temporary.

A pregnant woman is at a higher risk of having type 2 diabetes, once she is older than thirty years old.

Does not eat an excess of sugary food, prior to pregnancy

Type 2 diabetes develops because of high carbohydrate or high sugar diet. If a pregnant woman has been observing this type of diet before pregnancy and has a high level of glucose in her blood; she may not be suffering from gestational diabetes, but type 2 diabetes. This is more likely if she is age thirty or older

Previously gave birth to a baby weighing more than eight pounds

Women who have given birth to a baby weighing eight pounds or more, have a higher risk of developing gestational diabetes, unless the size of the baby is offset by the genetics of the parents.

Studies show that as a baby receives the same nutrients as the mother, it also acquires the high glucose level in the mother's blood, while in the womb. The increase in the glucose level may cause them to grow abnormally.

Was born with macrosomia.

Women who are born with the condition - macrosomia (i.e. she weighed more than eight pounds when born), are prone to gestational diabetes and type 2 diabetes.

Symptoms of Gestational Diabetes

Gestational diabetes has no symptoms, apart from the presence of sugar in your urine. If there are, they can be overshadowed by the changes in the body, during pregnancy. Therefore, it can be difficult to suspect you have the condition.

However, if you fit any of the characteristics described above, you should consider checking your blood sugar every month, during pregnancy. A fasting blood sugar (FBS) is more accurate than a routine blood sugar test. If you need an FBS test, you should fast for at least five hours, but no more than eight. If you have a routine blood test, it should be taken at least an hour after your meal.

You should inform your obstetrician, if your FBS test is higher than 7mmol/L. If you had a routine blood test, a level of 11mmol/L result could be a sign of gestational diabetes.

Complications of Gestational Diabetes

Untreated gestational diabetes may be temporary and reversible, but it can be dangerous to both the mother and child.

Possible complications of unmonitored gestational diabetes are:

- **High blood pressure**

  Pregnant women should have normal blood pressure, especially when nearing childbirth. Gestational diabetes can affect the blood pressure of pregnant women and cause it to fluctuate to critical levels. This could lead to an aneurysm or pre-eclampsia during child birth.

- **Edema**

  Gestational diabetes lowers the level of albumin (protein) in the blood. Albumin stops water or fluids escaping from blood vessels. If the level of albumin is low, fluid may escape and get trapped in other organs of the body. This fluid usually settles on the feet, making them swell. However, in some cases, fluid may settle in the brain and the lungs, which is dangerous and may be life threatening.

- **Ketoacidosis**

This rarely happens to women with gestational diabetes. However, when it does, it can be more dangerous to the baby than the mother. One study showed, that ketoacidosis during the first trimester of pregnancy may cause unintentional abortion; and malnutrition to both the mother and baby.

- **Macrosomia**

The fetus grows abnormally large in the uterus. It causes the baby to weigh significantly more than the average. About ninety per cent more than expected for gestational age. Depending on the mother's health and size of her uterus, macrosomia may result in premature birth and/or a caesarian section.

- **Type 2 diabetes**

This usually occurs if a woman, diagnosed with gestational diabetes, maintains a high carbohydrate and high-fat diet after the birth.

- **Difficulty breathing (for the babies)**

Gestational diabetes may cause the baby to have underdeveloped lungs. This can cause respiratory distress syndrome in babies, which makes it difficult for them to breathe. This condition is life-threatening, for babies under twelve months of age.

- **Hypoglycemia**

Babies born to a mother with unmonitored gestational diabetes may experience hypoglycemia during the first few weeks after their birth. This is due to the normal defense mechanism of the baby's body. They produce more insulin to balance the blood glucose level.

Some Guidelines for Women with Gestational Diabetes

A woman diagnosed with gestational diabetes can do the following, to help reverse or control it.

- **Avoid food with simple sugars**

  Cake frosting, soda, powdered juice and candies are high in simple sugars. Eating them will drastically increase the sugar level in your blood.

  Obstetricians, do not recommend lowering the carbohydrate and fat intake of a pregnant woman, as they are important during pregnancy. They recommend the woman gets her carbohydrate and fat from healthier sources.

- **Always monitor your blood sugar**

  Some women wait until they feel the symptoms of high blood sugar, before they get their blood sugar checked. If a pregnant woman waits, until they feel extreme hunger, thirst or drowsiness before their blood sugar is checked, complications may have already arisen in their body and their baby.

  It is important that women ensure they regularly monitor their blood sugar levels. Make sure you for further investigation at the first sign of a problem.

  Doctors often give a mother a schedule for prenatal checkups and mothers often only visit on that day. However, any abnormal symptoms should always be checked by her doctor.

  Delaying treatment of gestational diabetes may result in health problems for the baby and mother.

- **Exercise.**

  Exercise may help increase the sensitivity of the body to insulin. Pregnant women are limited to certain types of physical activity, but there are exercises specifically aimed at pregnant women. If the pregnant woman does not have time to take these classes, a twenty-minute walk before 8:00 am can help balance the level of glucose in both the baby and mother. Walking may also help lower the risk of preeclampsia.

Treatment for Gestational Diabetes

Oral medication may be prescribed to pregnant women. Doctors can also prescribe insulin injections, as a treatment for gestational diabetes, if levels fluctuate a lot.

Since these treatments can affect the growth of the baby, they must be given with care. The insulin injections used for mothers, will be pure human insulin, so it does not affect the development of the baby.

Prediabetes

The condition when your blood glucose level is higher than normal; but lower than the level for a Type 2 diabetic, is known as prediabetes.

When a person has a fasting blood sugar level of 5.6mmol/L to 6.4mmol/L, they may be considered prediabetic. A routine blood sugar level, with a result above 11.1mmol/L may also be considered prediabetic.

People with prediabetes are at higher risk of developing type 2 diabetes. However, this type of diabetes is reversible. Reversing it will help you prevent type 2 diabetes.

Who may become Prediabetic?

Prediabetes may happen to anyone, regardless of age. But, the following people have a higher risk of developing pre diabetes:

- Those who are overweight or obese

- Those who rarely exercise; or do any physical activity

- Those who were overweight or obese when they were younger

- Women who had gestational diabetes;

- Those with a family history of type 2 diabetes;

- People who don't eat healthily.

Symptoms of Prediabetes

Research has shown that the following symptoms of type 2 diabetes, start during the pre diabetic stage:

1. Acanthosis Nigricans or dark patches: Doctors suggest a blood sugar test should be taken at the first sign of darkness around the neck, or abnormal darkness in the knee and elbow region, regardless of the age of the person.

2. Hair thinning or hair loss: This is a tricky symptom, as many conditions may result in hair thinning and hair loss. But, if the person is obese, passive and eats a lot of sugary food, this could be a symptom of prediabetes or a start of type 2 diabetes.

Complication of Prediabetes

Prediabetes does not result in any health complication but may lead to type 2 diabetes; or gestational diabetes for pregnant women.

Treatment for Prediabetes

Treatment is not prescribed for people who are prediabetic. Experts recommend a healthy lifestyle to reverse it. If a pre diabetic continues to follow the lifestyle that reversed their prediabetes, they may not necessarily go on to develop type 2 diabetes.

Chapter 7

22 Myths About Diabetes

The scientific world knew about diabetes, as early as 1889 but there are still several myths surrounding the disease. These can perpetuate unhealthy practices that may lead to more problems. Here are some myths to be aware of if you or a loved one is diagnosed with the condition.

Myth 1: Diabetes is only caused by eating too much sweet food

Fact: Diabetes is not just caused by eating too many sweets. It is caused by a malfunction in the pancreas—type 1 diabetes, or hormonal imbalances that make your cells resistant to insulin— type 2 diabetes.

In fact, sweet food is not the only food you need to monitor, if you have diabetes, or you want to minimize your risk of developing it. You need to monitor your carbohydrate intake because in its most basic state, carbohydrate *IS* sugar. This means eating bread, rice, and pasta could prove to be just as harmful as eating chocolate and candy.

Myth 2: Diabetic people should not eat carbohydrate, or sugar at all

Fact: Carbohydrate is an important nutrient for the body, as it needs it for energy. It should not be completely avoided, even by diabetic people. What diabetic people need to avoid is eating high amounts of carbohydrates and sugar—more than their body can process. Your dietary requirements depend on your weight and your level of physical activity.

For example, eating a bar of chocolate may not be a concern for a reasonably fit man, who trains for a marathon or plays basketball every day. However, eating a single spoonful of ice cream may not be advisable for a person whose blood glucose level is 16mmol/L, especially if they don't engage in physical activity.

Myth 3: Type 2 diabetes only affects overweight or obese people

Fact: It is true that overweight or obese persons have a higher risk of developing type 2 diabetes. However, not all overweight or obese persons *will* acquire type 2 diabetes. Also, thin, or people with a healthy weight may develop diabetes. A healthy weight only lowers your risk of developing the disease.

Myth 4: Diabetes will go away once you achieve a healthy weight.

Fact: Apart from gestational diabetes and prediabetes, other types of diabetes do not go away once you reach a healthy weight. Diabetes is not tied to your weight, but is tied to how your body reacts to insulin.

However, having a healthy weight does increase your sensitivity to insulin, and allow you to manage the condition. Nevertheless, it will not get rid of diabetes once it has developed.

In fact, this is one of the reasons type 2 diabetics lose weight upon acquiring diabetes. Barring other variables, such as an increase in calorie consumption, they tend to lose weight on their own. It is a mechanism to balance the glucose.

Myth 5: Exercise is only advocated for type 2 diabetics. Type 1 diabetics should engage in minimal exercise.

Fact: Whether you are type 1 or type 2 diabetic, or even if you are not diabetic at all, you need to exercise. For diabetics however, their level of exercise needs to match their carbohydrate intake, to offset the glucose in their bloodstream. The less exercise or physical activity you engage in, the fewer carbohydrates you should consume.

N.B: You must exercise caution. If you exercise too much and do not balance your carbohydrate intakes, this may result in hypoglycemia.

Myth 6: Women who are diabetic may have difficulty having a child.

Fact: Diabetic women often have polycystic ovarian syndrome (PCOS), which makes it difficult for them to produce eggs or to conceive. A direct connection to diabetes, however, has yet to be proven. Some experts believe women with PCOS have a higher risk of acquiring diabetes; but diabetes plays only a minor role in the occurrence of PCOS.

Myth 7: All diabetic pregnancies result in macrosomia.

Fact: Diabetes only increases the risk of macrosomia. It does not mean that all pregnant woman, with diabetes will have a baby with macrosomia; and therefore, must undergo a cesarean section to give birth.

So long as the woman's blood glucose level is monitored during pregnancy; and carefully treated when it fluctuates, the pregnancy may not result in macrosomia.

Myth 8: Diabetes weakens your immune system

Fact: Diabetes only makes people feel drowsy and weak, when their blood glucose is at a critical level. It does not weaken the immune system. Also, having a healthy immune system will not always mitigate the chance of developing diabetes.

If the diabetic often contracts flu, cold or coughs, it is not due to diabetes; but because the immune system has been weakened for another reason. However, if these illnesses cause tissue damage, they may take longer to heal, if the person is diabetic.

Myth 9: Diabetes is a death sentence. A diabetic's life expectancy is lowered considerably.

Fact: This is no longer true. Experts studied diabetes and its complications in depth. It is easier to monitor and manage the disease than fifty or a hundred years ago.

A diabetic can still have good life expectancy if they manage their diabetes well.

Myth 10: You should become vegetarian or vegan, when you are diagnosed with diabetes.

Fact: Vegetarian and vegan diets do not have a direct effect on managing diabetes. Eating fruit and vegetables may be good for a diabetic, but the effects of the condition still depend on the amount of carbohydrate in a certain fruit and vegetable.

Eating too many high carbohydrate fruits and vegetables is not good for a diabetic.

Myth 11: Since insulin therapy is now available for type 2 diabetes, changing your lifestyle is no longer necessary.

Fact: Insulin therapy is to force your cells to react to, and stop resisting insulin. It should still be accompanied by a healthy lifestyle. If your blood continues to have a high level of glucose, the cells could still end up resisting insulin, rendering the insulin therapy ineffective.

Myth 12: Medications for Diabetes weaken and destroy the kidneys.

Fact: Diabetes itself weakens and destroys the kidney—not the medication. People may have this idea, because kidney failure often happens around the time doctors prescribe a higher dose of diabetic medication to patients. Nephropathy is a complication of diabetes. The diabetic medication is only an attempt to stop it.

Myth 13: Drinking a lot of water prevents you developing diabetes.

Fact: If you continue to consume excess sugar, therefore adding more glucose into the bloodstream, you may still develop diabetes. Drinking a lot of water will only ease or prevent the dehydration you experience because of diabetes. Dehydration is a result of your body's reaction to excess glucose. The kidneys use water to flush out the excess glucose, in your system, in your urine. The less water you drink, the more difficult it is for your kidneys to flush out the excess glucose.

Myth 14: Women with diabetes, always develop vaginal yeast infections (Thrush.)

Fact: Women with diabetes have a higher risk of having a vaginal yeast infection, but it does not mean they *will* have one. A diabetic woman, who observes good vaginal hygiene, may prevent the development of yeast infections.

Myth 15: Women with diabetes always develop vaginal stickiness.

Fact: A woman's urine may become thick, if she is taking any glucose inhibitor medication for her diabetes. This does not create a sticky feeling in the vagina, unless the woman is nearing her period. Again, it all depends on the woman' level of hygiene.

Myth 16: Kids diagnosed with type 1 diabetes may recover.

Fact: Type 1 diabetes is a chronic condition; and the person must live with it, usually for life. If the patient was under 10 years old, when they were diagnosed, there is no possibility they will recover.

Many type 1 diabetics, diagnosed at a very young age, become accustomed to a lifestyle that helps manage their blood glucose level. They incorporate it into their everyday life. It may appear to outsiders that they have got over their type 1 diabetes, as they do not let it limit their lifestyle.

Myth 17: All people that have a high level of blood glucose, when tested, are diabetics.

Fact: Not all people who have a high blood glucose level, when tested, are diabetic. There are occasions when a person's blood glucose level can increase drastically, but it is not considered diabetes.

Stress and sleeplessness may cause their blood glucose level to increase for a limited time. Treatment using steroids may also increase the blood glucose. However, these instances are still not considered normal.

According to studies, if these conditions occur to a non-diabetic person, it could mean they are at higher risk of developing type 2 diabetes.

Myth 18: Diabetes will lead to the slow deterioration in your health.

Fact: Diabetes, when properly controlled and managed, does not limit your life or necessarily cause other health issues. In fact, many diabetic patients, who manage to control their diabetes, express that the only difference between them and nondiabetic patients is their diet.

Myth 19: If you don't experience symptoms, you do not have diabetes.

Fact: In type 1 diabetes, you will experience symptoms. It is different with type 2 diabetes; and some patients may not feel, or be aware of any symptoms. They only discover their condition when their blood glucose is tested.

Some diabetic patients may think their doctor has made a wrong diagnosis because they have not experienced any symptoms. But, this could be attributed to the patient's ability to tolerate the symptoms.

Myth 20: Eating bitter melon can lower the blood sugar level.

Fact: Bitter melon contains a substance called "Charantin," which may help to lower blood glucose. However, research has shown that the amount of Charantin in bitter melon is not sufficient to lower the blood glucose levels effectively. A diabetic would need to eat 600 grams to 1000 grams of bitter melon, to try and control their blood glucose level for the day.

Myth 21: It is better to have hypoglycemia than hyperglycemia.

Fact: Neither of them is good; and experiencing either condition is cause for alarm. Both can cause dangerous complications to the body.

It may be quicker to give first aid for hypoglycemia as the treatment works faster, but then its effect also occurs faster.

Hyperglycemia may take longer to cause complications; but a sudden plunge in glucose levels, due to treatment with insulin, can still be dangerous.

Myth 22: Insulin therapy may cause a loss of vision.

Fact: Insulin is a lifesaver for diabetic people. Regardless of what type of diabetes a person has, it does not cause vision loss. This myth started as insulin therapy used to be the last recourse for many patients; and vision loss had already begun to occur, when treatment with insulin started.

Chapter 8

Prevention & Management Strategy 1

Constant Monitoring

According to experts, the best way to prevent type 2 diabetes developing is to observe the healthy lifestyle of someone who already has the condition, and is trying to manage it.

Diabetic people are encouraged to maintain a healthy lifestyle; and of course, this is also true for non-diabetics.

The only difference being, the diabetic may have to take medication to manage their blood glucose levels.

They should also make other lifestyle changes, such as avoiding smoking and drinking too much alcohol. It's also important to manage stress.

Below are the foundations of diabetes management

- Frequent blood glucose level testing/constant monitoring

- Maintaining a healthy weight, through exercise and diet

How Often Should You Check your Sugar Levels

Diabetes can be unpredictable. When symptoms of hypoglycemia and hyperglycemia appear, it usually means something has already gone wrong and the issue must be addressed fast. However, you should not just take diabetic medication, without knowing which you have.

If a diabetic uses insulin, they should test their blood glucose level at least 4 times a day. It is also recommended they undergo a fasting blood sugar (FBS) test at least twice a month.

For type 2 diabetics, it is recommended they check their blood glucose level at least once a day and have FBS test once a month. It is also recommended that they monitor their blood pressure at least twice a day.

You will need the correct tools to monitor your health; and this is discussed in detail, in the next section.

Equipment a Diabetic Should Invest In

Doctors used to have to monitor blood sugar levels and treat diabetic complications in their clinic or in the hospital. Today, it can be done by the patient at home.

Experts believe it is important diabetics are aware of what to expect with their disease; how to monitor their condition at home, and how to treat complications when they arise. It could help save their life; and could also save time and money, as they don't need to have the tests carried out in a clinic or hospital.

Diabetic equipment has also become affordable and therefore, easier to invest in.

Diabetics are encouraged to have their own equipment, so they can monitor their blood sugar level. This could help avoid dangerous complications. They also need a first aid kit, to treat themselves until medical help arrives, if required.

Below are some equipments a diabetic should invest in:

1. **Glucometer or blood glucose meter**

   This is used for routine blood sugar monitoring. Every diabetic should have one at home, along with glucose strips.

   The result you get from a glucometer is not as accurate as the one you get from an FBS. However, it is accurate enough to tell you whether your blood sugar is at an abnormal level, or not.

It is wise to choose a glucometer that can be operated with one hand. This makes it easier to check a blood sugar level, independently and anytime/anywhere.

2. **Lancets and glucose strips**

A glucometer is of no use unless these are also present, especially the glucose strips.

Use only medically approved lancets, because regular needles or syringe needles may cause deeper wounds, which could cause complications in a diabetic.

Each brand of glucometer will usually have it's own specific brand of glucose strip. So, make sure to buy the correct type.

3. **Blood Pressure monitor or sphygmomanometer**

For younger type 1 diabetics, a blood pressure monitor may not be necessary. But, if a diabetic is over thirty, it is recommended they have their own blood pressure monitor, regardless of the type of diabetes they have.

Fluctuations in sugar level may also affect blood pressure. So, older diabetic patients should monitor their blood pressure, as often as they monitor their blood sugar levels.

A digital sphygmomanometer is highly recommended, as they are easier to use unaided and the results are available quicker.

4. **Blood sugar and blood pressure record book**

Diabetics are often required to keep a record of their blood sugar level and blood pressure level, especially if they are still adjusting to a diabetic lifestyle.

A regular notebook and pen will do; or there are also journals made for these, which may be available free with other diabetic supplies. Some digital glucometer and sphygmomanometers can store at least 100 results.

5. A small box of hard candy

Diabetics should always have some hard candy at hand. Hard candy is the first line of treatment for hypoglycemia; and is more effective than soft candy, as it releases sugar slower.

6. Weight scales

Though weight scales will not be used as often as other equipment, it is still advisable that diabetics have their own. Fluctuations in blood sugar level can be triggered by weight gain or loss.

7. Insulin and syringe kit

Type 1 diabetics need to have a constant supply of insulin, needles, syringes and sharps boxes. Insulin needs to be stored in a cool place; so, having a thermal insulin kit will keep the insulin cool for a while, if they are out for the day.

8. Ketone strips

These are necessary for type 1 diabetics, but are rarely needed by type 2 diabetics. The strips measure the level of ketones in the body. They can tell whether a patient is suffering from ketosis or ketoacidosis. Ketosis is milder; while ketoacidosis may be a life-threatening situation for a diabetic. Thus, having the ketone strips at hand is recommended.

Chapter 9

Prevention & Management Strategy 2

Attaining and Maintaining A Healthy Weight

Please Note - Most diabetics are under the care of a Specialist at a hospital. They will arrange for you to see a dietician to help you get your diet under control. They can also refer you to the physiotherapy team, and they will give you the correct "safe" exercises to undertake, Exercise should be correctly monitored and increased gradually, especially if you are obese. If you want to lose weight, and/or want to start an exercise regime you must always have a check-up with your doctor first. What follows is a guide to help inform that journey.

Being slender or muscular does not guarantee a person is at a healthy weight. This depends on the person's body mass index (BMI) i.e. the ratio of the person's weight in proportion to his/her height.

An overweight person weighs more than 10% of their ideal BMI, but not more than 20%. A person who weighs more than 20% of their ideal BMI, is considered obese.

How to Calculate Your BMI

To calculate your BMI, divide your weight in kilograms, by your height in meters squared.

For example, if Adam weighs 75 kilos (approximately 165 lbs.) and has a height of 1.2 meters (a little less than 4 feet) to calculate his BMI, the equation would be:

$$\text{BMI} \quad 1.2\text{m} \times 1.2\text{m} = 1.44\text{m}^2$$

$$75\text{kg} / 1.44\text{m}^2 = 52.08$$

If you live in the United States, where the Imperial measurement system is in practice, use online converters that are available.

What is the Normal BMI?

Underweight	Less than 18.5
Normal weight	18.5 to 24.9
Overweight	25 to 29.9
Obese	30 or more

Therefore, in the example above, Adam would be considered extremely obese.

The higher a person's BMI, the more likely they are to develop diabetes and cardiovascular diseases.

Weight Loss Guide for Diabetics

It is safer and more beneficial that everyone maintains a healthy weight. There are two phases to achieving a healthy weight, especially if you are a type 2 diabetic. The first phase is to lose the excess weight and the second is maintaining a healthy weight. Both tasks are not easy, but the second phase can be harder than the first.

Losing weight naturally may be more difficult, but is preferred, over resorting to surgical intervention; which obviously comes with its own risks. The principle behind natural weight loss is calorie deficit but this should be combined with physical activity. Therefore, the calories that go into your body should be less than the energy needed to use them up. This way, your body will start to use stored fat for energy.

Eating a Low-Calorie Diet

85% of diabetics are obese or overweight and 70% of these are also physically inactive. If a diabetic person eats a high-calorie diet, they need more physical activity to burn the calories. However, please note, it is dangerous for an obese person to start strenuous exercise suddenly.

To make it possible for diabetics to lose weight, without drastically increasing their physical activity, they need to *lower* their calorie intake.

The daily calorie consumption, for an average person, should not exceed 3000 for males and 2500 for females. It should not usually be lower than 1800 for men and 1200 for women.

For a diabetic, trying to lose weight, it is advised that their new "normal" is 1800 calories for men and 1200 calories for women. This ensures they can still perform exercise or other physical activity.

However, weight loss through diet should be made gradually. A sudden drastic drop in calorie intake may cause shock to the body's organs, which can result in their own health complications.

Engaging in More Physical Activity

Boosting physical activity enables a person to avoid making drastic changes to the number of calories they consume. The more a person moves, the more calories they burn. As a result, they start to lose weight and benefit from the bonus of endorphin release, which improves mood.

Increasing physical activity should always be done gradually, whether it is for a diabetic or a non-diabetic. This is necessary for the protection of the heart. Make sure you undergo a physical checkup before undertaking any exercise routine.

Experts recommend a daily exercise routine. However, if you can't find enough time for the gym, or working out at home, changing how you do a few things can help.

- *Walk, jog or ride a bicycle to work*

  According to a study, walking a mile continuously can help you shed up to 100 calories, in 30 minutes. A brisk walk can help you lose up to 180 calories a day. If you jog, then you lose more. Jogging at a speed of 5 miles per hour can help you lose about 240 calories, every 30 minutes. Cycling enables you to lose 180 per 30 minutes.

- *Wash clothes by hand*

Washing 5 kilograms of clothes enables you to lose 75 to 120 calories. If you do not want the detergent to ruin your hands or skin: Try rinsing your clothes three times and hanging them outside on a clothes line, instead of using the dryer. You could lose 30 to 50 calories!

- *Mop or scrub the floor manually*

  Instead of using an electric steam mop, 30 minutes of mopping or scrubbing the floor, may help you lose 120 calories.

- *Wash your car yourself*

  By washing a sedan for thirty minutes you can potentially lose up to 180 calories. This includes the actual washing and drying of the car. If you add polishing, you can lose another 30 calories.

- *Play a physical game with your children*

  According to experts, this is better than organised exercise. A short 30-minute playtime with your children, which may include a game of tag or shooting hoops, can help you lose at least 220 calories. The reason you lose more calories doing this is the stress-free factor. According to some studies, smiling while doing an activity may make you lose 20 calories, but laughing while doing an activity may make you lose 40 to 60 calories, every 30 minutes.

Ideal Weight Loss Rate for Overweight Diabetics

This topic is the subject of ongoing debate among experts. Some say a type 2 diabetic should lose weight as fast as possible, while others say it should be done slowly. Many believe however, that it depends on how obese the person is.

If the patient is extremely obese, they need to lose weight more rapidly. The longer a diabetic remains obese, the more quickly complications may arise. However, if the patient is merely a little overweight, they can take it more gradually. The body will automatically force itself to lose weight, as a defense mechanism to balance the level of blood glucose.

However, doctors advise that regardless of how overweight a diabetic is, it is best not to lose more than 5.44kg (12 pounds) a month. To lose more than this, would require the diabetic to eat less than 1200 calories a day, which can also be detrimental to their condition.

Steps to Correct Weight Loss

- **Establish how overweight you are**

  You do this by obtaining your BMI. This will determine how much weight you need to lose.

- **Determine your ideal weight**

  You can do this by multiplying an amount ranging from 18.5kg (40.78lbs.) to 24.9kg (54.89lbs.), which is the ideal BMI, with the amount equivalent to twice your height.

  Say you choose 24.9kg and your height is 1.65 meters.

  To find a person's ideal weight, the equation would look like this:

  Ideal weight   1.65m + 1.65m = 3.3m

                        24.9kg x 3.3m = 82.17 kg (181lb.)

- **Determine how much weight you need to lose**

  To do this you need to subtract your ideal weight from your current weight. This provides the amount of weight you need to lose.

  For Example: Current weight   100.00kg

                      Ideal weight   82.17kg

                      You need to lose   17.83 kg

- **Set a time scale for your weight loss**

  Since the recommended maximum amount of weight loss per month is only 5.44kg (12 lbs.) you will need approximately 14 weeks to lose 17.83 kg (39 lbs.)

- **Determine the average calories you need to subtract from your day**

  You need to do this to achieve your target weight loss for the month.

  To do this, keep in mind that 0.45kg (1lb) is equivalent to 3500 calories. Multiply 3500 by a number of kilograms you want to lose and you will get the total calories you need to lose in a month. Then, divide this result by 30.

  For example, you need to lose a total   17.83kg (39lb)

                                                                   17.83kg x 3500 = 62,000 calories/month

                                                                   62,000/30 days = 2,066 calories per day

  This means you need to burn an extra 2,066 calories in a day.

- **Determine how much exercise you need for a day**

  You need to subtract the calorie you need to lose from the maximum calories a person should have in a day.

  If you are a woman, subtract it from 2500. Subtract it from 3000 if you are a man.

  Since the maximum calories a person should have in a day should not exceed 2500 (for women) or 3000 (for men), then using the example in No' 5 you would only be left with a calorie intake of 434 and 944 respectively.

However, dropping the calorie intake to these numbers is extremely difficult, if you are used to eating far more than the daily-recommended values. You can make this easier by adding exercise into the mix.

N.B: Your dietician will come up with a diet, specifically tailored to you. Please seek their advice. This is to give you the idea of diet/exercise principle.

- **Choose your diet to exercise proportion**

  How many calories do you want to lose by exercising and/or by dieting? Knowing your daily physical activity can help with your decision.

  ➢ If your physical activity involves doing light household chores and sitting at a desk for work or school, you may only be burning 80 to 120 calories for those tasks each day.

  ➢ If your physical activity involves 30-minutes jogging and aerobics, then you might be burning 200 to 300 calories for those tasks each day;

  ➢ If your physical activity involves major household chores, heavy training jobs and vigorous sports exercise, you may be burning 400 to 600 calories for those tasks each day.

  For example: Wendy needs to lose 1200 calories. She works as a teller at a bank, and does not have enough time to do major chores at home or exercise. We can assume Wendy will only lose about 100 calories, each day, for her physical activity.

  For example:

Wendy needs to lose	1200 calories/day
She already burns	100 calories/day
She needs to burn a further	1100 calories/day

Should she increase her physical activity more or should she remove calories from her diet?

Wendy decides to lose 800 calories through dieting

Then she can lose the other 300 through exercise.

Maintaining a Healthy Weight

Maintaining weight is more difficult for type 2 diabetics, as they must exercise twice as hard to lose weight.

Humans do not always lose weight in a linear manner. If you continue to follow the routine you have developed, by following the steps to losing weight, your weight could plateau, or increase even if you stick to a strict diet. This is due to the body's natural defense mechanism.

If a person continues to follow the same strict routine to lose weight, their body will go into starvation mode as a defense mechanism. It is afraid it might lose too much weight. It will try to store fat, causing weight gain. According to researchers, after 6 to 8 months of following a routine to shed 4.53 to 5.44kg (10 to 12lb.) a month, they should modify his routine.

Many experts believe the best way to maintain a healthy weight, upon achieving it, is to increase calorie intake by at least 20%. However, this amount should not exceed 1800 calories. You then need to offset the additional calorie intake by increasing physical activity. The body does not go into starvation mode, if it loses calories through exercise but when it loses calories by the loss of nutrients.

So, if after six months, Wendy achieves her healthy weight, she should consider changing her routine.

Based on the example in the previous topic, Wendy is planning to take 1700 calories a day. She may need to increase her calorie intake to 2040 calories after six months. Since there are an additional 340 calories in her diet, Wendy may need to add more exercise, or add any physical activity that will help counteract these calories.

Chapter 10

Prevention & Management Strategy 3

Exercise Routines

A diabetic should consult with his/her physician before taking part in any exercise routines. There are routines or activities that may not be safe for diabetics. A person with prediabetes may not have a limit to any exercise routines, provided they have no other ailments.

6 Exercise Routines for Diabetics

Below are some popular exercises that a diabetic may be able to do:

Jogging

A thirty-minute jog, every day, can help lose at least 240 calories daily. Aside from losing calories, it also helps strengthen ankle and leg joints. It also helps prevent neuropathy in the legs. Moving the legs often, may also reduce the risk of edema in the feet.

It improves the circulatory system and strengthens the cardiovascular and respiratory system.

Aerobics

Thirty minutes of aerobic exercise burns about 180 to 240 calories; and has the same benefits as jogging. However, an obese diabetic needs to be very careful. If they have not done this type of exercise before, they must do it gradually. Some exercise routines put a lot of pressure on the legs, which can cause injury to obese people.

Swimming

A thirty-minute swimming can help you lose 210 to 360 calories, depending on your speed. This is a good exercise for the lungs and the heart. In fact, many experts claim it is the best exercise for diabetics. It helps to burn calories quickly and doesn't put pressure on the joints.

Ball Games, e.g. basketball, volleyball, football

Engaging in these sports for thirty minutes can cut 180 to 270 calories. These sports can help burn more calories, as they are usually played with others, which helps increase the "feel good factor."

Shadow kickboxing

You would need to be already fit to undertake this exercise. However, it can help to shed more calories. At least 300 for thirty minutes. It not only helps you lose weight, but tones your muscles.

Diabetics with heart ailments or chronic respiratory ailments might still be able to do this type of exercise, but they would need to do it lightly and with the approval of their doctor.

Yoga

An hour of basic yoga moves can help you lose about 280 calories. Routines that specifically target certain areas of the body may help you lose a few more calories.

Yoga is considered a good choice for diabetics, as it improves blood circulation. It also relaxes the body, but awakens the sensitivity of the nerves.

Types Of Exercise To Avoid

A pre diabetic person can try these exercise routines, but for those with chronic diabetes, some exercise poses a dangerous risk.

Body building exercises

Using weights during exercise is not dangerous, and in fact may be recommended, but there are limits.

A diabetic person should not lift weights that are so heavy they put a strain on their muscles. This could worsen diabetic neuropathy. Lifting heavy weights also put extra pressure on the eyes and nerves of the diabetic. This could damage the small vessels and cause the nerve to become numb.

Adversarial contact sports

Doing shadow-contact sports can be good for a diabetic, but actual contact sports *are* dangerous. Diabetics heal more slowly than healthy people. If they are injured or wounded during the match, they may develop further complications.

8 Exercise Safety Measures

A diabetic should always be prepared when they are working out. Doing physical activity without careful preparation may cause complications or at worst, life-threatening situations.

Ensure you do the following prior to exercising:

5. **Eat at least one hour before exercising**

   A diabetic should not carry out any physical activity on an empty stomach. It increases the risk of hypoglycemia and ketoacidosis.

   Eat a light snack, prior to exercising. Many diabetics prefer to exercise an hour after breakfast.

6. **Always carry water and hard candy**

   Diabetics are usually thirstier than healthy individuals, especially during exercise. It is important they have water at hand, to counter dehydration.

   Having your box of hard candies with you, may prevent you from a sudden hypoglycemic attack.

   Hard candy is seldom required by a type 2 diabetic, but it does no harm to have them there in case hypoglycemia occurs.

7. Check your blood glucose level before exercising

Vigorous physical activity or exercise can make the body react in two ways. It Can cause sugar levels to drop, which is the usual reaction for type 1 diabetes. With type 2 diabetics it could cause sugar levels to rise.

So, before undergoing any exercise, a diabetic should check their glucose levels. If their level is below 5.5mmol/L, the diabetic should consider eating something sweet before exercising. However, it is probably best to refrain from rigorous exercise.

If the blood sugar level is above 15mmol/L, a diabetic should not take part in any rigorous exercise. Their high blood sugar may go higher due to exercise.

8. Check your blood pressure

This is necessary for type 2 diabetics, although Type 1 diabetics over twenty-five years old are also advised to do the same. Exercise increases the blood pressure; and it is dangerous for a diabetic to exercise when their blood pressure is high.

9. Protect your feet

Diabetics needs to know how their feet will be affected, by the exercise or the physical activity they are planning to undertake. They need to protect their feet from injury.

Be careful when choosing shoes for exercise. Make sure they support the ankles and won't cause blisters.

10. Do not exercise an hour after you have had your insulin injection

The effect of insulin usually peaks an hour after it was injected. This means the blood sugar level will drop. Exercising at this point can be dangerous, as the exercise will also lower the blood sugar levels. This will result in a hypoglycemic attack.

11. Don't exercise alone

Whatever exercise you choose, do not do it alone. Having a friend or family member present during exercise can help if an emergency arises i.e. a hypo or hyperglycemic attack

12. Never ignore your body's signals

Stop or do not exercise, as soon as you feel any symptoms of hypoglycemia, hyperglycemia or hypertension. If it occurs post exercise, consider doing a ketone test, glucose test and blood pressure test. If the level of any of the tests is abnormally low or high, seek medical attention immediately.

Exercise routines can do wonders for your health. Just keep safety in the forefront of your mind when engaging in any physical activity.

Chapter 11

Prevention & Management Strategy 4

Diabetic Meal Plans

Many nutritionists believe the diet followed by diabetics is a good diet for everyone. Anyone who follows it lowers their risk of developing diabetes and other health conditions.

Many diets have claimed to be the best for diabetics. A few examples are: a ketogenic diet; a vegan or vegetarian diet; a Mediterranean diet; or other diets that have a low carbohydrate and low glucose intake. However, which is the best for diabetics? This chapter is dedicated to answering this question.

5 Characteristics of a Diabetic Diet

Experts say that the ideal diabetic diet has the following characteristics:

- **It is low in calories**

  Diabetics should eat a low-calorie diet, as opposed to a low carbohydrate diet, especially type 2 diabetics. Lowering calories means you lower the actual amount of carbohydrate and fat you need to burn.

  Low-carbohydrate and low-fat diets may not work for diabetics, as they may then increase proteins in the digestive tract and the bloodstream to a dangerous level. Diabetic people, especially those with type 2 diabetes should not consume a large amount of protein, as it may increase their risk of neuropathy and other complications. If the amount of fat and carbs, in the diet, is significantly decreased, while the amount of protein remains at a proportionate level, the diabetic may suffer from malnutrition. Thus, the solution is to lower overall calorie intake.

- **The amount of carbohydrates should not be less than 45%, but no more than 60% of the total calorie intake each day.**

  These levels of carbohydrates (45% to 60%) are considered the safe amount for a diabetic to consume.

  If a diabetic observes an 1800-calorie daily allowance, the number of carbohydrates he/she eats should be within 810 to 1080 calories.

  For pregnant and breastfeeding women, the amount should not be less than 50%.

- **The amount of protein should not exceed 1 gram, for every 0.45kg of his/her ideal weight, and no lower than 0.4 grams.**

  Diabetic patients, especially those with type 2 diabetes, should not consume too much protein. It may worsen their nephropathy and make them more prone to dehydration.

  Previously, nutritionists suggested the protein intake of diabetic patients should be 15 to 20% of their total calorie-intake for the day. However, it has recently been discovered that the amount of protein should be proportionate to the weight of the person.

- **The amount of fat in a diabetic's diet should not be more than 25% of the amount of the ideal total calorie allowance for the day.**

  Some dieters often allocate the remaining amount of the "ideal total calories" each day to fat. So, if the remaining amount is 35%, that would be the amount of fat in their diet.

  Many experts disagree. The percentage of fat should be low, especially if the person is over twenty-five years old. Too much fat, whether from a good source or not, can still lead to complications, such as heart disease and hypertension. Also, it interferes with insulin receptors, causing glucose levels to rise.

- **Their diet should have less fried and processed food.**

  Fried and processed foods are high in unhealthy fat and refined carbohydrates. They increase the level of glucose in the blood, blocking insulin receptors and increasing cravings for sweet and greasy food.

  Foods that retain their natural flavor are usually high in fiber and low in sugar. Fiber aids digestion and helps "choose" which nutrients are absorbed, or not, by the body.

How To Calculate Your Daily Carbohydrate, Protein and Fat Requirements (5 Steps)

Using the characteristics of a diabetic diet, we can calculate the ideal amount of carbohydrates, proteins and fat needed for a balanced diet. Here is a step-by-step approach to balancing the type of food in the diet.

Step 1: Know your ideal weight.

The formula to work out your ideal weight is discussed in the previous chapter.

Step 2: Choose your ideal total calorie intake for the day.

To work this out, follow step 5 of "steps in losing weight" in the previous chapter.

Step 3: Calculate how much protein you need in calories.

Since proteins must be proportional to your weight, it is better to calculate this first. Multiply your ideal weight by an amount within 0.4 to 1 gram per pound. Multiply the result by four.

Step 4: Calculate the amount of carbohydrates.

The ideal amount is usually somewhere between 45-60%. It should be proportional to the degree of the person's physical activity. If they are very active, they could consume as much as 60%.

Step 5: Allocate the remaining amount to fat.

This should not exceed 25%. The remaining amount of calories can be allocated to fat. However, if the level of fat exceeds 25% of the total calorie intake, then the ideal total calorie intake should be lowered.

For children under seventeen years of age, the amount of fat can be increased to 30%.

To illustrate, consider the example below:

Wendy's ideal weight is 120 pounds. Her ideal total calorie intake for the day is 1800. She prefers to eat 0.5 grams per pound. Since, she is a bank teller and has low physical activity, she chooses to consume carbohydrates equivalent to 45% of the total calorie intake. To balance her diet, she would have to consume:

- 240 calories of protein
- 810 calories of carbohydrates.
- 450 calories of fat (based on the maximum of 25%)

Wendy can only consume 1500 calories a day, using this calculation, instead of 1800.

Now, Wendy may choose to adhere to this new calculation or increase the amount of carbohydrate or protein.

Converting Grams to Calories

Most food manufacturers on the market list their product facts using grams. It is enforced by states, but also a marketing strategy. The number of grams is smaller than the number of calories. If a consumer sees the product only has 15 grams of fat, he might not be too worried. However, if they see the product contains 135 calories from fat, they might think twice.

Ignoring these totals is not an option for diabetics. They need to be more vigilant in knowing how many grams/calories they consume each day. They must convert the weight in grams to calories. Knowing this helps to them to arrange the correct meal plan for the whole day.

Some might think that this is too complex. However, diabetics do not always have to calculate the calorie value for each food. Diabetic associations often supply dietary guides that include conversions.

If you cannot find a manual, you can do it using the table below:

1. 1 gram of carbohydrate is the equivalent of 4 calories.

2. 1 gram of protein is equivalent to 4 calories.

3. 1 gram of fat is the equivalent of 9 calories.

Using the example of Wendy above, her diet for the day should be composed of food with the following weights:

- 60 grams of protein. That is 240 calories divided by 4.

- 202.5 grams of carbohydrate. That is 810 calories divided by 4.

- 50 grams of fat. That is 450 calories divided by 9.

Getting Macronutrients from the Right Source

Another vital aspect of a diabetic plan is choosing the source of your food. A diabetic may be eating the correct amount of protein, carbohydrates and fats, but if they are coming from a bad source, his/her diet will not be healthy.

According to nutritionists, diabetics should source their carbohydrates, fat and protein from *natural and unrefined foods.*

Processed foods may contain the same amount of nutrient, but they break down into synthetic chemicals that may be harmful to the body.

Types Of Food To Eat & Those To Avoid

1. Carbohydrates

When choosing carbohydrates, you should always try to eat those from unrefined sources, whether you're a diabetic or not. Unrefined sources have higher amounts of dietary fiber and do not break down into simple sugar.

Good Sources of Carbohydrates	Sources of Carbohydrates that should be avoided or limited
• Whole grains, such as corn, wheat, oats, brown rice, and quinoa.	• White rice, white bread, pasta made from refined grains
• Fresh fruits, those with lesser juice, like avocado, berries and pears are preferred • Fresh vegetables, especially green leafy vegetables and those from squash family	• Dried and preserved fruits and vegetables. • Diluted fruit juices
• Fresh milk	• Powdered milk • Processed milk
• Freshly cooked beans, lentils and other legumes	• Preserved beans and other legumes

2. Sugar and Sugar Substitutes

Another bad source of carbohydrate are sweeteners, such as table sugar. You may only be consuming a small amount, but they increase the glucose level in an instant. However, you do not need to eliminate them from your diet, but you must limit them.

Products like honey, molasses, brown sugar, coconut sugar and stevia are claimed to be safe for a diabetic person. There are no studies or approved research that prove this fact. The only proven fact is that these products break down slower than refined white sugar. The body absorbs them slower and hence, they do not have such a drastic effect on the body. Thus, experts still advise diabetics to use them sparingly.

Experts recommend using natural sweeteners found in fruits and vegetables. If a sweetener must be used, honey e.g. manuka honey is preferred, because it is lower calorie and has other health benefits.

3. Fat

There are many good sources of fat, but processed fat has become the most accessible. Some products claim to be low in fat or nonfat, but they have hidden and dangerous types of fat.

For example: A bread company may advertise their whole-wheat bread to be low-fat. However, the fat they used to make the bread may be processed. Therefore, it can be argued it contained a large amount of unhealthy fat.

There are four types of fat. These are:

- *Polyunsaturated fat*

  Omega 3 and Omega 6 are examples of polyunsaturated fat; they help to control cholesterol.

  Aside from lowering cholesterol and reducing the risk of heart diseases, they also aid in cell growth. New cells help improve the way glucose is received and therefore, reduces the risk of developing diabetes; or having uncontrolled diabetes.

  Sources of polyunsaturated fat include flax oil, sunflower oil, almonds, avocado and oily fish e.g. mackerel.

- *Monounsaturated fat (MUFA)*

MUFA also controls cholesterol in the body; reduces the risk of heart disease and the risk of developing diabetes, or uncontrolled diabetes. MUFA retains its liquid form, unless it is chilled.

Good sources of monounsaturated fat are olive oil, avocado, nuts, sesame seeds and fish.

- ### *Saturated fat*

    Many people think saturated fat is unhealthy fat. Nutritionists claim that all fats are good fats, even saturated fat. However, it is consuming too much that is bad for your health.

    Studies show saturated fat helps lower the blood sugar in the body, as it helps increase the body's sensitivity to glucose. However, if the amount of saturated fat consumed exceeds 6%, it can cause complications by increasing the level of cholesterol in the bloodstream.

    Sources of saturated fat include butter and coconut oil.

- ### *Trans fat-or hydrogenated oil.*

    Trans fat is unhealthy for diabetics, and even to non-diabetics. Almost all unnatural and processed food contains trans fat. Do not be deceived by "0-gram" claims on the labels. Companies often claim a product has "0-gram" trans-fat, when it does contain trans-fat – it is just that the amount does not exceed 0.5 grams. Therefore, eating a large amount of food that claims to have "0-gram" trans-fat might still make you consume a lot of trans fat.

    Foods high in trans-fat are processed French fries, cakes, muffins, margarine and shortening.

4. Protein

Protein is required for building and repairing tissues. It is also essential in the production of hormones and other nutrients. It helps in the production of insulin, which is also a type of protein.

Plant-based proteins are a healthier source for diabetic patients, than animal-based. The former is more efficient in producing hormones and other nutrients essential for the body, and they also contain fewer calories.

Nuts, soybeans, legumes and kale are good sources of plant-based protein.

For animal-based protein, fish and free-range, lean meat is a good source of protein.

Distributing your Daily Calorie Needs

Knowing how many grams you need and the type of food to fulfil your daily calorie needs is only one side of the equation. The second part of planning is dividing your daily calorie needs among your meals.

One suggested approach is that you reduce the size of your meals as nighttime approaches. Specifically, you should:

3. Eat a heavier breakfast;

4. Eat a moderate lunch;

5. Eat a light dinner/supper.

However, some believe this rule is not acceptable for all diabetics; and in fact, many experts state this approach is only suitable for prediabetics. It is not advisable for type 1 diabetics, as they may suffer from hypoglycemia while they sleep, due to the lack of carbohydrates.

Recommended schedule of meals

A more acceptable schedule is eating five small meals a day, with sufficient interval between meals. Below is one recommended schedule of meals for a diabetic.

- **Breakfast should not be more than twelve hours after supper.**

  Some dieticians may disagree with this. Blood sugar levels could drop to dangerous levels if the person fasts for more than 10 hours. However, some doctors and experts still recommend a twelve-hour interval between supper and breakfast.

  A diabetic is advised to drink a glass of milk before bedtime, to avoid hypoglycemia.

- **Snacks should be between two to three hours after meals (Breakfast and Lunch.) Snacks should not be skipped, even if the diabetic does not feel hungry.**

  Diabetics often complain of hunger two to three hours after eating a meal, when in fact, they are not hungry. It is the body sending a misleading signal to the brain and other organs. If the diabetic ignores these signals, the body wants to defend itself and the organs try to protect themselves from hunger by *conserving* energy. Diabetic complications may arise as a result of this. So, doctors suggest eating a small amount of food, regularly. This helps produce enzymes that convince the body it is not hungry.

- **Lunch should not be more than 6 hours after breakfast.**

  Diabetics should on no account skip lunch, especially type 1 diabetics. Diabetics need a regular intake of carbohydrate to maintain their blood sugar level. Skipping lunch or any meals may trigger ketoacidosis.

- **Dinner/Supper should be more than 6 hours, but not more than 10 hours from lunch.**

  Supper is just as important as breakfast, for diabetics. The body needs a store of carbohydrates and fat, for the body to process while it is asleep. If there is nothing to process, it can trigger hypoglycemia and in some cases for type 1 diabetic, ketoacidosis.

Step by Step Guide to Distributing your Calories to Each Meal

Here are the steps to help you allocate the number of calories for each meal:

- Divide your ideal daily calorie needs into four.

  Though you need five meals a day, you only need to divide your total calorie needs into four because one portion is divided into two snack portions.

- Let's assume your ideal daily calorie needs are 1800. Then, each meal should be approximately 450 calories, with two snacks of 225 calories.

- Calculate how much carbohydrate, protein, and fat do you need for the day. For this, we would use the plan we calculated for Wendy:

    o 240 calories of protein

    o 810 calories of carbohydrates.

    o 450 calories of fat

- List what you would like to eat for each meal. A diabetic diet does not limit your choice, but ideally it needs to be healthy, unrefined and within your daily calorie allowance.

    For example, you may want to eat:

    Breakfast - 2 scrambled eggs, 2 slices of whole-wheat bread and a cup of coffee

    Lunch - A large bran chicken sandwich for lunch and 1 cup fresh tomato juice

    Snacks - ½ cup of berries and 1 apple

    Dinner/Supper - T-bone steak and green salad with lemon vinaigrette for dinner

- List the carbohydrate, and fat and protein for each meal. Taking the example above, let's assume that:

The breakfast totals 418 calories

Carbohydrate:	192 calories /48 grams
Protein:	100 calories/25 grams
Fat:	126 calories/14 grams

The lunch totals 470 calories

Carbohydrate:	220 calories/55 grams
Protein:	124 calories/31 grams

Fat: 126 calories/14 grams

The snacks total 129 calories

Carbohydrates: 112 calories/28

Protein: 8 calories/2 grams of protein

Fat: 9 calories/1 gram

The supper totals 328 calories

Carbohydrate: 88 calories/22 grams

Protein: 96 calories/24 grams

Fat: 144 calories/16 grams

Tabulate everything. Compute the total of the calories, grams of fat, protein and carbohydrates. The tabulation for the above example, would result in the following:

Total Calories for Each Meal	Carbohydrates for each meal (Cals)	Protein for each Meal (Cals)	Fat For each meal (Cals)
Breakfast: 418	192	100	126
Lunch: 470	220	124	126
Snacks: 129	112	8	9
Supper: 328	88	96	144
Total 1345	**612**	**328**	**405**

Compare the meal total planned with your ideal distribution. You need to check whether your meals fit within your ideal calorie distribution.

In the tabulation above, the carbohydrate is *less* than the required amount, while the protein is *above* it. So, does this fit within your ideal calorie distribution?

If you base it purely on the numbers, you would have to say "no". However, if you consider the fact that the values we used are based on Wendy, who is 54.4kg (120lb.), the distribution is still balanced.

The total calories do not fall below 1200.

The value of protein 328 calories is still within the limit for the daily protein requirement (1g per pound).

The fat does not exceed 450 grams.

The only problem is the carbohydrate. It is below 45%, or is it? Nutritionists suggest setting an allowance, when you are planning a calorie based diet. It's likely you will be using mass produced ingredients, especially spices and seasoning.

Many of these products often contain hidden fats and carbohydrates. The manufacturers may not declare the correct amount/type of carbohydrates or fats, to make the calorie levels appear lower. So, in this case, the deficit of 258 calories may possibly be compensated for by hidden carbohydrate from the bread and sauces used for the meals.

What if the amounts in your tabulation are too low, or too high, compared to the ideal distribution?

The planned meal is too low from the ideal distribution, if it falls below 1000 calories. It is too high, if it exceeds 2500 calories.

Falling or exceeding your ideal calorie distribution for one or two days may not cause problems but, doing so on a regular basis often causes complications.

If your actual calorie intake is significantly lower, then the diet is not providing the correct nutrition your body requires. This could result in malnutrition, frequent weakness, and frequent hypoglycemia.

If it is significantly higher than the ideal calorie distribution, it will not control blood sugar levels and increase the risk of diabetic complications.

In chapter 11 there are a few recipes to help prevent diabetes developing or for taking control of your diabetes. The recipes have the corresponding calorie values, which make it easier for you to adjust the portions depending on your calorific needs.

Chapter 12

Breakfast Recipes For Diabetics

Berry Oatmeal

Ingredients:

- 4 cups low-fat milk

- 2 cups of regular rolled oats (not quick cooking)

- 1 cup blueberries, raspberries or mix

- 2 tablespoons honey, raw (optional)

Direction:

1. Brown the oats in a deep pot, placed over medium heat.

2. Add the milk and cook the oats over a low heat. Stir constantly to avoid burning the oats at the bottom of the pot.

3. When the oats are cooked, remove from heat and add the berries.

4. Break some of the berries to release their juice.

5. Add the honey, if desired.

6. Serve.

Nutritional Information:

Servings: 6

Total Calories: 232

- Carbohydrates: 92 calories

- Protein: 85 calories

- Fat: 55 calories

Egg Sandwich

Ingredients:

- 1 whole egg
- 2 slices of whole-wheat bread
- ¼ cup avocado, cubed
- Lettuce leaves
- Salt and pepper to taste
- ½ teaspoon olive oil
- 1 teaspoon vinegar

Directions:

1. Place a skillet over low heat. When warm, add the oil.
2. Crack the egg into the skillet and scramble quickly until set.
3. Add salt and pepper to taste and mix again.
4. In a separate bowl, mash the avocado and mix in the vinegar.
5. Spread the mashed avocado on the lower layer of bread.
6. Place the lettuce leaves over the avocado; and then place the egg on top.
7. Top with the second layer of bread.

Nutritional Information:

Serving: 1

Total Calories: 417

- Carbohydrates: 172 calories
- Protein: 92 calories
- Fats: 153 calories

Banana Pancakes

Ingredients:

- 2/3 cup whole-wheat flour
- 1 cup all-purpose flour
- Pinch of salt
- 2 tablespoons of white sugar
- 2 1/2 teaspoons baking powder
- 1 1/2 cups buttermilk
- 1/2 cup ripe bananas
- 1/4 teaspoon olive oil

Directions:

1. In a bowl, combine all the dry ingredients.
2. Lightly mash the bananas and add them to the dry ingredients.
3. Gradually add the buttermilk until you reach a batter-like consistency.
4. Place a pancake grid or a nonstick pan over a low heat.
5. Grease the pan lightly with olive oil.
6. Scoop 1/4 cup of the batter and place it in the hot pan.
7. Cook for about 2 minutes on each side, or until both sides are brown.

Nutritional Information:

Servings: 6

Total Calories: 193

- Carbohydrates: 160 calories
- Protein: 24 calories
- Fats: 9 calories

Apple Quinoa Porridge

Ingredients:

- 1/4 cup quinoa
- 1/4 teaspoon cinnamon powder
- 1/2 cup water
- 1/4 teaspoon nutmeg powder
- 1/2 cup diced apple
- 1 teaspoon raw honey
- 1 teaspoon chia seeds

Directions:

1. Boil quinoa, cinnamon powder, nutmeg and water for 1 minute over medium heat.
2. Lower the heat and simmer until the quinoa is tender. This will take approximately 10 to 15 minutes.
3. Mix in the rest of the ingredients. Cool a little before serving

Nutritional Information:

Servings: 1-2

Total Calories: 264

- Carbohydrates: 200 calories

- Protein: 28 calories

- Fats: 36 calories

Vegetable Frittata

Ingredients:

- 1 onion, chopped
- 1/4 cup diced button mushrooms
- 1 red pepper, chopped
- 1 stalk asparagus, chopped
- 5 egg whites

- 3 whole eggs
- 1/3 cup non-fat milk
- 1 cup Cheddar cheese, grated (optional)
- Olive oil, as needed

Directions:

1. Sauté onions in a pan, over low heat until caramelized. Add the remainder of the vegetables.
2. Grease a glass baking dish and pour in the vegetable mixture. Spread over the base of the pan.
3. Beat the egg whites, whole eggs and milk. Add a pinch of salt
4. Pour the egg mixture over the vegetables. Tap the pan to make sure that some of the egg mixture gets to the bottom of the dish.
5. Spread the grated cheese on top.
6. Place in a 160 ^{0}c preheated oven and bake for 20 minutes.

Nutritional Information:

Servings: 4-6

Total Calories: 223

- Carbohydrates: 32 calories

- Protein: 56 calories

- Fats: 135 calories

Lunch and Dinner Recipes

Pan-Fried Tuna with Pineapple Salsa

Ingredients:

- 4 180-gram tuna steaks (salmon or other fish may be used)
- Salt and pepper to taste
- Juice of 1/2 lemon
- Olive oil, about 1 tablespoon
- Salsa
- 1 cup fresh pineapple, chopped finely

- 1 cup of mix red and green peppers
- 1 cup cooked corn kernels
- 1/4 cup onions, sliced
- 1 teaspoon chilli peppers, sliced
- 1/4 cup orange or lime juice
- 1/2 teaspoon cumin
- 1/4 cup parsley

Directions:

1. In a bowl, combine all ingredients except for the tuna, 1/2 lemon, and olive oil. Mix thoroughly and chill for at least an hour.
2. Season the tuna with salt and pepper. Pour lemon juice over the tuna.
3. Heat a nonstick pan over medium heat. Pour in a little olive oil.
4. Cook the tuna for a total of 5 to 10 minutes (Treat similarly to steak.) Depending on the tuna steaks thickness, and to desired taste.
5. Place a 1/4 cup of salsa over the tuna before serving.

Nutritional Information:

Servings: 4

Total Calories: 455

- Carbohydrates: 261 calories
- Protein: 140 calories (35 grams)
- Fats: 54 calories

Broiled Salmon with Brown Rice

Ingredients:

- 4 180-grams salmon

- 2 to 4 oranges

- 2 teaspoons crushed peppercorns

- 2 teaspoons vinegar, preferably apple cider or red wine vinegar

- Green onion or leeks, about 1/4 cup, optional

Directions:

1. Preheat the broiler.

2. Slice the oranges into 1/4-inch rounds and arrange half of them in the bottom of a broiling pan.

3. Season the salmon, with peppercorns and vinegar.

4. Arrange the remaining orange on top.

5. Broil for 15 minutes.

6. Serve with brown rice.

Nutritional Information:

Servings: 4

Total Calories: 256

- Carbohydrates: 112 calories

- Protein: 108 calories (27 grams)

- Fats: 36 calories

Beef and Vegetable Stir Fry

Ingredients:

- 500-grams sirloin steak, sliced thinly

- 1 cup broccoli, in small florets

- 1/2 cup carrots, julienned

- 1/2 cup red pepper

- 1/2 cup onion

- 1 tablespoons olive oil

- 2 tablespoons light soy sauce

- 1 teaspoon brown sugar

- 1/2 tablespoon peanut butter

Directions:

1. Combine the peanut butter, 1/2 teaspoon of brown sugar and the soy sauce in a bowl.

2. Place a nonstick frypan over medium heat, and sauté the onions in olive oil until caramelized.

3. Add the sirloin strips and cook for 2 minutes.

4. Stir in the rest of the vegetables and cook for another 2 minutes.

5. Pour the peanut butter mixture and mix. Cook for another minute.

6. Taste. Add a bit more sugar if needed.

Nutritional Information:

Servings: 4-6

Total Calories: 264

- Carbohydrates: 56 calories

- Protein: 120 calories (30 grams)

- Fats: 153 calories

Chicken Whole-Wheat Pasta

Ingredients:

- 300 grams whole-wheat pasta, cooked according to instructions

- 200 grams of chicken breast, broiled and diced

- 1/2 onion, chopped

- 1 16-ounce can of diced tomatoes, or 3 cups of diced fresh tomatoes

- 2 tablespoons of Italian seasoning, or you can use 1 tablespoon of basil, 1/2 tablespoon of oregano and 1/2 tablespoon of parsley with 1/2 teaspoon cumin

- Salt and pepper

- 1/4 cup Parmesan cheese, grated

- Olive oil, about a teaspoon

Directions:

1. Place a large nonstick pan over medium heat. Add a few drops of oil and sauté the onion until it is translucent in color.

2. Add the chicken and fry for about a minute.

3. Add the diced tomatoes and the Italian seasoning and cook for 7 to 10 minutes.

4. Season with salt and pepper.

5. Pour over the cooked pasta. Toss and serve.

Nutritional Information:

Servings: 4 to 6

Total Calories: 137

- Carbohydrates: 104 calories

- Protein: 60 calories (15grams)

- Fats: 18 calories

Low-Fat Chicken Tenders

Ingredients:

- 1 kilo of chicken breast fillets

- 1 cup fresh pineapple juice

- 1/2 cup packed brown sugar or 1/2 cup honey

- 1/3 cup light soy sauce
- Sliced chilli peppers, optional

Directions:

1. Cut the chicken fillets into strips. Then thread them onto skewers.
2. In a bowl, combine the other ingredients.
3. Arrange the skewers in a pan and pour over the marinade. Set aside for an hour.
4. Grill on both sides for 5 minutes or until the juices of the chicken run clear.
5. Serve over any of the following: steamed brown rice, quinoa, couscous or with a bowl of fresh green salad.

Nutritional Information:

Servings: 10

Total Calories: 182

- Carbohydrates: 22 calories
- Protein: 124 calories (31 grams)
- Fats: 36 calories

Macronutrient Conversion Table

To help you make your own meals or to check the nutrient content of your favorite recipes, here is a short table of the macronutrient content of some common ingredients.

Ingredients	Fat Grams	Protein Grams	Carbohydrates Grams
1 hard-boiled egg	6	7	2
1 cup of roasted almonds or cashews	45	27	18
Apple Pear Peaches Pineapple	Less than 1 gram	Less than 1 gram	12 grams average
1 cup avocado	22	3	13
1 medium Banana, 1 medium	Less than 1 gram	2	23
Blueberries, raspberries, and other wild berries	Less than 1 gram	1	15
1 cup of brown rice (cooked)	1	2.6	23
1 tablespoon of butter	12	Less than 1 gram	Less than 1 gram
Chicken breast, roasted or grilled	3.5	31	1
1 cup of couscous (cooked)	Less than 1	3.6	23

1 tablespoon of honey	Less than 1 gram	Less than 1 gram	17 grams

100g Kale
 	
   Broccoli
 	
   Cauliflower
 	
   Beet
 	
   Spinach
	Less than 1 gram	7 grams average	8 grams average

100g Lentils	Less than 1 gram	9	21
Lettuce Carrots	Less than 1 gram	2 grams average	10 grams average
1 cup Low-fat milk (1% fat)	2	8	12
1 cup Milk (whole)	8	8	12
1 tablespoon Olive oil Flaxseed oil	14	0	0
Peanuts, roasted 1 cup	50	26	14
1 cup Quinoa (cooked)	3.6	8	39
1/2 cup of red and black Kidney beans	Less than 1 gram	12	60
180g Salmon (grilled or broiled))	12	35	Less than 1 gram

100g Scrambled eggs	11	12	6
180g Sirloin steak	22	43	Less than 1 gram
100g slice of sponge cake (plain)	4.3	7	58
Strawberries	Less than 1 gram	1	11
Sweet potato Potato	Less than 1 gram	2 grams average	20 grams average
180g T-bone steak	24	42	Less than 1 gram
100g of tofu	5	8	2
180 g tuna (grilled or broiled)	10	43	Less than 1 gram
100g or 2 slices of whole-wheat bread	3	13	41
1 cup of plain yogurt	2	9	41

*Most other fruits and vegetables have less than 10 grams of carbohydrate; and less than 1 gram of fat and protein.

Conclusion

I hope this book has provided informative information about diabetes; how to minimize your risk of developing it, or if you have the condition to help you to control it. More importantly, I hope this book had also encouraged you to live a healthier lifestyle.

Do not let the disease control your life. Enjoy your life; just remember to eat healthily and avoid smoking and heavy drinking. You can still enjoy the occasional "guilty" pleasures, but you need to restrict their consumption.

For those living with a diabetic person, I encourage you to embrace their lifestyle. It will provide them with moral support and encourage you to live a healthier lifestyle. It may even reduce your risk of developing the disease.

For parents of children with type 1 diabetes, please note this book is mainly aimed at adult diabetics. Though the basic principles may be applicable, I still encourage you to check with their pediatrician before trying any strategies in the book.

Thank you again for downloading this book. I wish you a healthy life.

The End

Thank you very much for taking the time to read this book. If you found this book useful please let me know by leaving a review on Amazon! Reviews are the lifeblood of independent authors. Your support really does make a difference and I read all the reviews personally so I can get your feedback and make this book even better.

If you did not like this book, then please tell me! Email me at BarbaraTrisler@yahoo.com and let me know what you didn't like. Perhaps I can change it. In today's world a book doesn't have to be stagnant, it can improve with time and feedback from readers like you.

You can impact this book, and I welcome your feedback. Help make this book better for everyone!

Thanks again for your support!

	Books By Barbara Trisler	
Book #	**Book Title**	**Learn More**
1	Air Fryer Cookbook For Beginners	Link
2	Air Fryer Cookbook For Beginners With Colour Pictures	Link
3	Paleo Diet Cookbook For Diabetics	Link
4	Paleo Diet Cookbook For Diabetics With Colour Pictures	Link
5	Air Fryer Cookbook For Beginners (2nd Edition)	Link
	The kindle edition will be available to you for FREE when you purchase the paperback version from Amazon.com (The US Store)	

Lightning Source UK Ltd.
Milton Keynes UK
UKHW030631050221
378309UK00011B/798